View from the Cliff

A COURSE IN ACHIEVING DAILY FOCUS

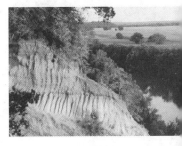

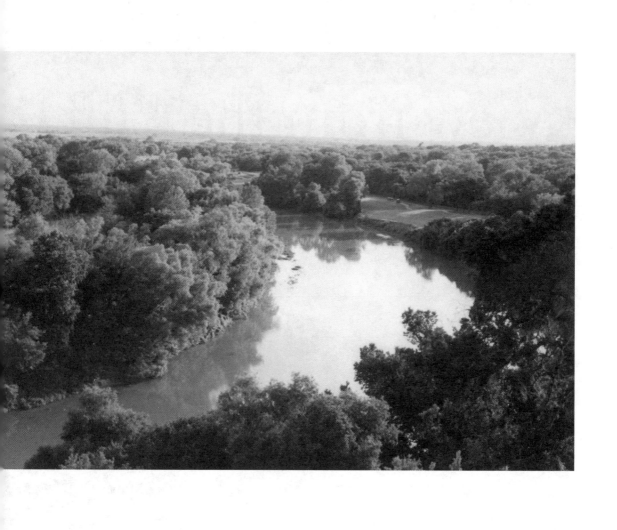

View from the Cliff

A COURSE IN ACHIEVING DAILY FOCUS

Lynn Weiss, Ph.D.

TAYLOR TRADE PUBLISHING

Lanham • New York • Toronto • Oxford

Published by Taylor Trade Publishing
An imprint of The Rowman & Littlefield Publishing Group, Inc.
4501 Forbes Boulevard, Suite 200
Lanham, Maryland 20706

Distributed by National Book Network

Designed by Barbara Werden

Library of Congress Cataloging-in-Publication Data

Weiss, Lynn.

    View from the cliff : a course in achieving daily focus/ Lynn Weiss.

      p. cm.

   ISBN 0-87833-253-7 (pbk.)

    1. Attention-deficit disordered adults. 2. Attention-deficit hyperactivity disorder. 3. Self-esteem. I. Title

RC394.A85 W447 2001

616.85'89—dc21   00-051075

Printed in the United States of America

ACKNOWLEDGMENTS

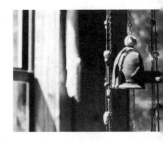

Writing *View from the Cliff* is the culmination of many years of work that has seen ADD (Attention Deficit Disorder), the disorder, transformed into a style of brain construction whose attributes reflect as many assets as negatives. I have come to realize that many people who would never be "diagnosed" with ADD do, in fact, deal with daily issues that are dependent on a style of brain construction that is creative, expressive, lively, kinesthenic (learning by doing), and feelings based.

Throughout this process many people have helped me see and capture this perspective.

My editor, Camille Cline, hung in there with me as we bridged brain style differences with grace and respect.

The Taylor Publishing Company staff—Jim Green, Sales Director; Barbara Werden, Art Director; Anita Edson, Publicist; Diana Shaw, Special Sales; and all the others—helped assemble all the elements.

View from the Cliff has benefited greatly from my work at the Federal

Correctional Institution, Bastrop, Texas. The staff and inmates have allowed me to try out many of these strategies. Special thanks to: Janice Taylor, FCI teacher, who first introduced me to the prison; Leah Parrish, Educational Supervisor, who welcomed me and allowed me to take as much learning away as I brought to the institution; and John Rubel, PhD, Psychologist, who built bridges with case managers, drug and alcohol counselors, and the psychology department.

Personal support has come from my adult children, who continue to support their mom; my dog, Candy, who agreed to be photographed for the cover and has kept me company through the writing and rewriting of every word in this book; and the wonderful friends who make my life full.

CONTENTS

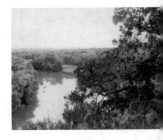

View from the Cliff

A COURSE IN ACHIEVING DAILY FOCUS

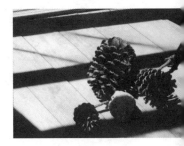

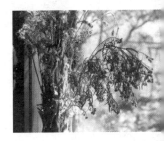

INTRODUCTION

A young man in prison khakis walks toward me down a dimly lit hall. We're in the education building of a low-security prison.

Even before I can clearly see his features, I notice his swagger. Every part of his body moves as he walks. His head tosses errant hair back from his forehead, his arms churn, his hips sway, and his gait proclaims loudly that he is on a mission.

"Hmmmm," I think, assessing what I see. His silent bravado proclaims his inner sensitivity and insecurity about our scheduled meeting. None of this is new to me in this setting. "Am I to be trusted?" is the critical first thought in any first-time meeting that takes place in prison.

I reach out my hand and say, "Hi. You're Titus, aren't you? I'm Lynn Weiss." The twenty-year-old takes my hand almost reluctantly but quickly responds to my firm, sure grip. It is as if, in the flash of an eye, he sees something he can trust in me—maybe just a little.

His GED teacher referred Titus to me because he was "driving her nuts." Seems he moves his chair close to the wall and tilts it backwards so he can rock back and forth while he attempts to do his studies. When she tells him to put all four legs of the chair on the floor, he does it . . . for about five seconds, and then the next thing she knows he's tilting backwards and rocking again.

He is teetering on the edge of getting himself thrown into the "hole." That means he is in danger of being locked up twenty-four hours a day in a tiny cell that will cause him to miss school and work from which he earns money. He'll also lose "good time," which will delay his release.

In 1998 I'd introduced an ADD skill-building group for inmates into the prison. The teacher was very aware of ADD characteristics and had decided to refer Titus both to the group and for individual work with me before writing him up.

"He's not a bad guy," she had told me. "Some are. He's not. He's young and not mean, but he's sure not learning. In fact, his GED pretest scores are plummeting instead of improving." Then, in an offhand comment, she added, "You know, he seems to do better work when he's rocking."

It made sense immediately.

With this in mind, I ask Titus, smiling, "What's the deal with your chair-rocking business?" Then, I add, "You know it's making your teacher nuts, and that's not good for her or you." With that I look him directly in the eye with a little twinkle showing in mine.

He flashes a smile, then a frown, and begins with a drawl, "Well . . . ." He hesitates.

I jump in and say, "Titus, look, whatever you say is confidential. I think you're a good guy, but there's some reason you keep doing what your teacher doesn't want and it's my job to figure out the reason. It will be your job to use what I find out so you can stop messing up and stay out of trouble. Okay? Got it?"

Titus nods and his bright eyes look straight at me. He understands.

"I'm not trying to hassle my teacher.

Mostly I don't even know I'm doing it."

"Mostly?" I query.

He grins. "Sometimes I do it on purpose when I'm bored."

I respond half seriously and half jokingly, "Whew, that's a high price for reducing boredom—if you keep it up and lose good time! But," I shrug, "that's your choice." My voice is nonjudgmental as I state a reality of prison life.

At that, Titus gets serious and says, "I don't want to get into trouble here. But I kinda feel it's hopeless. I'm trying hard, but no matter how much I want to do good, I do something like tilt my chair back when I don't even mean to do it. My pretest scores are even going down."

Over the next few weeks, Titus and I meet weekly, and he also attends an ADD skill-building group that teaches him how brain construction affects his behavior, his interests, and his ability to do his schoolwork. He learns many of the techniques included in this book. He proves to be an avid worker and quick learner. As a result he begins to be in control of achieving success.

Almost immediately Titus stops tilting his chair. Because he learns better when he's active, we focus on his learning to use alternative ways to move around while he is in class. He learns to break his assignments into manageable pieces. He discovers ways to keep his attention on his schoolwork. His pretest scores begin to rise.

Titus's swagger disappears, and he becomes less volatile when touched or surprised. He comes to understand his sensitivity, but he also practices ways to get what he needs while both protecting himself and staying out of trouble.

Three months later, his teacher reports, with a catch in her voice, that Titus has passed the GED exam. Word comes from the guards that he no longer causes trouble in the unit, mess hall, and rec yard. He is promoted to a better-paying job in prison industries. He begins to save the money he earns for when he is released. He's considering taking college-level correspondence courses. He's even beginning to think about what he might like to do when he is released from prison. Perhaps he will end up teaching others what he has learned. Time will tell.

Is Titus unique? No. In nearly fifteen years of group and individual work with adults with ADD attributes, I've heard the same story over and over and over with minor variations. I've watched the same outcomes unfold, person after person. By no means is Titus that unusual, whether he's behind bars or outside.

Part of what I've learned over these years is to look at ADD as brain diversity. I'm talking about a genetic style of brain construction that is simply a stylistic trait passed from generation to generation through a family line. I'm not talking about acquired attentional problems such as result from diet, head injuries, cocaine or alcohol abuse, metal poisoning, birth defects, or allergies.

I've seen many of us lose touch with the usefulness of our innate ADD style because our natural style didn't fit the expectations of the world around us. Titus, too, had resources that went unrecognized—resources that he could use to achieve his goals. Instead, feeling hopeless to get his studies *right* yet trying to get an education, Titus distracted himself by "misbehaving."

What Titus had to learn is what we all must learn. We must go about the job of discovering our inner resources. Then we must find ways to use them on our own behalf. Titus also had to discover ways to heal the feelings of hopelessness and helplessness that he had learned as a result of not being tuned into his hidden resources. These lessons make up the themes woven through this book.

Many of us no longer see our innate talents. We don't recognize and have not received appropriate training to use our natural skills and talents. We have underachieved and been hurt as a result, and we've often given up trying "to get things right."

The skills in this book were originally forged with people who have a high number of ADD attributes. I've come to realize, however, that many of the issues that emerged for them are issues many more people experience to some degree. Each of us must find out how our brains are made. We must be sure we find the right places to utilize those resources so we may use them positively. We must, above all, refine our thinking tools to accomplish outcomes that make sense for each of us and maximize our effectiveness.

Then, strong in our own right, we can team up with others who have a different constellation of skills. Together we become unbeatable.

How to Use This Book

You will find three themes woven throughout this book. Many of the suggestions are geared to help you recognize and support the innate brainstyle attributes with which you are born—the ones that reflect your greatest strengths.

But when your innate strengths are pressed into learning and living envi-ronments that don't fit them, you end up hurt. As a result you will need to find ways to heal those hurts so you can use your natural skills effectively.

Finally, you will discover ways to accommodate your natural skills and interests to situations that don't fit you. The trick here is to do what you need to do without damaging yourself in the process.

Theme One: Hidden Resources of The True You

You have a natural style of brain con-struction—one with which you are born. I call that style The True You. It is from the core of your true self that the hidden resources, previously dormant or disallowed, will be encouraged to come into full bloom. In this book, you will be encouraged and helped to recognize and respect your hidden resources. What lay previously undetected or underdeveloped can be embraced and used in your personal and work life for the benefit of all.

The True You is the unwarped, unjudged, unwounded, natural you. All of the original innate skills, talents, attributes, and gifts with which you were born are available to you to use as you choose. In this book, I'll ask you to focus on the way in which you think, act, and express yourself. I'll talk about what you like and how you can go about reaching the goals that are important to you in a way that fits your natural bent. I'll look at how to make use of your brain in ways that can provide you with both happiness and success.

You'll learn to recognize what fits you by noticing feelings of enthusiasm and hesitation within yourself. You will be drawn to activities and situations that are right for you, that support your natural skills, and that provide you with a sense that you can reach your potential. In contrast, you will begin to learn to recognize your hesitation to engage in activities and situations that don't naturally fit you and that are not good for you. As you honor this wisdom within yourself, your life path will smooth out. Your journey will belong to you. Your pleasure will increase. You will come to know meaningful success.

Theme Two: The Wounded You

No matter how you were raised or what your style of brain construction, you undoubtedly bumped into situations that did not fit your natural style of learning and working. You most likely felt bruised. As a result, you also probably learned to disregard your natural resources for learning and accomplishing things so that they went underground out of your conscious awareness.

The result means you have been hurt, though often unintentionally. You'll learn how you can heal those hurts. Then you'll be able to effectively reconnect with The True You. You'll become aware of the right environment for you—one that serves the needs of your true self so you can retrieve your lost skills and talents.

In today's world, there are three typical causes of injury that you are likely to have suffered.

■ *Socialization*—All societies have beliefs about what are right and proper ways for their members to behave. When these beliefs do not reflect the reality and diversity of how humans are made, wounding results. If, for example, sitting still in school is thought to indicate a high level of socialization, then those of us who learn by being active will be hurt. It's that simple.

■ *The Learning of Harmful Beliefs*— Wounding happens when a person believes there is only one acceptable way to be, to do, to think, or to live. All other ways, the result of different innate skills and talents, are considered flawed. Previously, beliefs have been the business of religion, but the damage done by beliefs has now spread throughout medicine, education, employment, and the legal system. Labeling ADD/ADHD (Attention Deficit Disorder/ Attention Deficit Hyperactivity Disorder) as a disability and placing it within the categories of the Americans with Disabilities Act is an example of such a belief.

■ *The Leveling of Judgments*—If a person with the untapped resources of the true self is judged to be pathological because his or her natural way of doing things doesn't fit the current social model, the person is wounded by virtue of being judged. This applies to people labeled with ADD/ADHD. They are even said to have a medical problem, are often denied an education that fits their brain construction, and are judged for work by standards that preclude their showing what they can do.

In addition to being thwarted from using their natural talents, they must be labeled *disabled* in order to be given an opportunity to achieve. Further damage comes from having to raise their hands and say, "There is something *wrong* with me."

SECONDARY WOUNDING

Further damage occurs when a person has bought into the belief that his or her innate way is wrong. Self-depreciation results and continues damaging a person as long as the belief persists.

If you are required to do something that doesn't fit you and you resist, complain, react, or become depressed, anxious, clumsy, or indecisive, you are likely to be scolded, chastised, or further labeled because you've reacted. When you resist, you may be called oppositional. When you complain, you may be called argumentative. When you cry or become depressed, you are called symptomatic. When you become anxious, you are given a pathological label and medication to deal with your symptoms.

But these secondary symptoms are only the result of being pressured or forced to do something that doesn't fit you in the first place—something that is out of alignment with what is in the best interest of The True You. Then when you are additionally labeled with behavioral or emotional problems, you are wounded a second time.

This latter wounding of people with diverse brainstyles does not need to happen. The secondary problems or symptoms are not inherently a part of the original true self. The behaviors and feelings are only indicators that something is amiss with the relationship between an individual's way and the environments in which that person is living. Instead of the person needing to change, the environments may need to be changed. The True You needs to be saved from being required to do what doesn't fit. Then the secondary symptoms disappear.

Theme Three: The Accommodating You

Even when you have mastered The True You and know the kinds of settings in which you can optimally function, you will encounter the imperfect world of everyday life. Living in an imperfect world means you will not always be able to find a fit between your natural ways and the environments you face. But you can learn skills to bridge the differences between your innate skills and the expectations placed on you. And you can do this without hurting yourself further.

ACCOMMODATING TO YOUR ENVIRONMENT

As you become aware of The True You, you will learn to recognize how well your surroundings fit you. You'll become attuned to beliefs that honor you. At the same time you will continue to respond the best you can until you can do something to make changes.

On a personal level, you will be able to make plans, aligning your life with the needs of The True You. But such moves take time. Take, for example, a move to self-employment. This will require time to adjust your finances, family obligations, and inner courage before you can actually make the step. You may also need to acquire some new skills. While you are acquiring the tools you need to make such moves, you will learn to accommodate to your current situation so you are not further wounded.

In this book, you will find both the light at the end of the tunnel and illumination as you travel to that light. Know that you are perfect the way you are naturally constructed. Know that your untapped resources are desperately needed not only by you but also by the society in which you live. But also know that there is usually a considerable lag between any new way to look at a situation and the actual changing of society to accommodate that new perspective.

The Rewards of Diversity

As you get to know yourself, your strengths and weaknesses, and what to do about them, you can become aware of what you need in order to allow those strengths to flourish. You become aware of which expectations and situations fit you and which don't. You then are able to make choices that are in your best interest. Once you're in tune with The True You, you'll begin to see a style of pursuit that fits you best as you strive toward a goal. Even when expectations upon you and requirements of a goal do not fit you, you'll be able to find ways to proceed that do not set you up for failure. You can rationally measure the differences between your natural self and the requirements of the situation and escape self-depreciation. You then learn to accommodate to situations that don't much fit you without being maimed in the process.

With perspective, you will no longer hold yourself to impossible expectations. Instead, you'll find pathways to achieve the outcomes you desire in ways that use your strengths. No longer do you need to be hounded by shame, guilt, and feelings of inadequacy. The prize will be the good feelings you have about yourself and successful utilization of the best of what you innately have to offer any situation.

Tools for the Journey

Natural Resources

Let's look at the skills that often go untapped in today's world. People with lots of creative, right-brained natural ability will recognize and feel at ease with these resources. Others with a more linear way of doing things may not wish to utilize them but may find knowledge of them helpful in recognizing how others see the world and approach tasks.

Either way, knowing what these resources are gives all of us a balanced palette of skills when we encounter brainstyle differences on our way to accomplishing goals.

- *We see the big picture*—Many of us see the big picture before we see or make use of any of the details that make it up. Usually creative by nature, big picture people often see a complete vision of what we want to achieve before we start moving toward our goals. In fact, we don't travel well to any goal unless we are provided with the big picture to begin with.

- *We think in terms of how things function*—If we are to know how to proceed toward a goal, we must know its purpose. How is this goal to be used? Rather than seeing the details that make up the task, we see the function the details play. Then we can know the steps to take to achieve the goal.

- *We pay attention to the patterns and relationships within the big picture*— Our focus of attention tends to be on the relationships between details rather than on the details themselves. We first see the interconnections and patterns that are formed between things rather than the elements that make them up.

- *We express high levels of activity, physical, mental, emotional, and verbal*—Naturally invested with lots of energy, we learn, create, and produce best when we are active. Our innate skills seek environments for expression that allow us to be physically active and verbally expressive. Our minds are curious and exploring and often work at lightning speed. After all, we see the big picture first, so we don't need to slowly progress from one detail to another in order to reach that completed picture. We're also aided by our rapid awareness of the patterns that often give us early clues about the journey we are taking. The icing on the cake is the presence of big, broad, expressive emotions that communicate to us and others with clarity.

- *We learn by doing (kinesthenic learning)*—We naturally learn *through* the process of doing something rather than by reading or listening *about* whatever we are learning. We write a book to learn to write. We don't learn to write a book by studying about writing a book, doing exercises or worksheets, or taking exams so we can then write a book. We are totally and completely able to learn any subject or body of professional material, no matter how complex, by utilizing kinesthenic learning. That's why the apprenticeship model works well for us.

■ *We have an inner locus of perception and control*—Our worldview comes from within ourselves. Our ability to organize, work with time and timing, maintain control over our behavior, and do whatever we need to do is idiosyncratically guided from within ourselves rather than from outside. We know and sense and can learn to live in a responsible way that yields the same results achieved by our more linear counterparts if we follow what feels *right* to us. We know what to do by listening to our inner drumbeat, not by using a template produced outside of ourselves into which we are expected to fit.

■ *We have a high level of sensitivity*— Our sensitivity is felt through our senses: sight, sound, taste, smell, and touch as well as intuition. Extremely empathetic, our sensors are calibrated finely. Liken us to the dog that hears sounds not perceived by the human ear. We sense at a level that not all people have available to them. We are empathic and responsive to our environments. We can be wounded when others do not see or sense the source of the wounding, yet we experience it nonetheless. When a companion has a feeling such as anger, we know it even if the person is unaware of it and denies it. Many of us are psychic though we may not be comfortable with this skill or may not purposely use it.

■ *We are responsive*—Because we are so sensitive and tend to act kinesthenically when attempting to reach a goal, we tend to be seen as reactive. With a wide range of emotions, readily experiencing joy and pain, we often express our feelings and do something about situations that others do not even know exist.

- *We have a strong sensing capability*—We tend to think first through our ability to sense what is going on rather than by thinking about something. We simply *know*, having an inner sensory vision, experience, or intuition. We often feel the sensing physically in our bodies. Once we've perceived an event on a sensory level, we can decide what to do in response. We even store information using this mechanism rather than by categorizing according to the labels in more general use.

- *We resonate to the rhythmic timing of nature*—Rather than responding to an arbitrary scheme to keep track of time, we tend to use natural rhythms and our own internal timing to get things done. We can apply this skill to a project or to getting the rest our bodies need. We may work at night and sleep in the daytime. We may naturally eat at times that vary from a three-meal-a-day schedule. We rarely break projects down into equal time segments in order to get them done by a certain time, but rather work when we *feel* creative and don't work when we feel unwilling or hesitant. When our innate timing is allowed to blossom and we are trained to recognize it, we always get things done *on time*.

Diversity

There is not one right way to be. There is a wide range of variation in the way in which humans are constructed. We all have our unique perspectives of life, shaped by our innate physical construction. Our bodies and brains look and function differently. Our experiences vary widely, so how in the world can we be expected to do things in the same way?

Each of us is born with certain strengths and limitations. One person is

Introduction

expansively creative while another makes detailed records of transactions. A third has characteristics of both and is able to bring the creative expressions into orderly presentation for all people to enjoy. No one style is better than another. Every strength has an up side and a down side. It is for each of us to realize what these strengths are in ourselves and to use them to advantage.

The honoring of diversity whether it is in relation to skin color, sexual identity, age, or brain construction is a must if we are to become healthy human beings and our society is to become one in which variation yields wholeness. In this context each of us plays a valuable role no matter how we are made. But before we can honor the diversity brought by variations in brainstyle, we must recognize both its existence and its value for the society as a whole. We must learn when to rely on our own skills and when to team with others to produce a broader outcome.

This book is dedicated to assisting each of us to be all we can be and to contribute the best we have to offer for the good of our society as we learn to achieve daily focus.

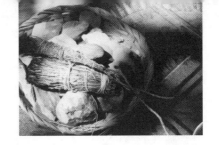

PART ONE

Organizing in New Ways

*In truth and with grace
it is now time to allow the
medium of the Self
to emerge.*

JAMIE SAMS
1990

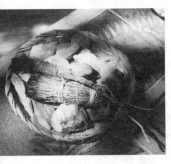

Everyone can organize, but we don't all do it in the same way. It doesn't matter whether we're talking about managing details, keeping track of volumes of numbers and letters, breaking projects into manageable steps that guarantee completion, or making efficient and responsible use of our time.

Yet the skills needed to accomplish these tasks elude many of us. As a result, we come to believe we are disorganized. And we are, when we try to organize in ways that don't fit us. As a result, questions arise such as, "What's wrong with me?" and "Am I not trying hard enough?"

To understand what's happening, let's remember the purpose of organization: to be able to retrieve things and manage a flow of work that will get us to a goal of our choosing. How we do it and what our process of organization looks like is not the issue. Given this freedom, we may discover we have a perfectly workable system. If, however, organization is supposed to mean alphabetized labels, file cabinets with papers out of sight, clean surfaces, and goals arrived at one step at a time, we may fail abjectly and be branded incompetent.

Our success at organization depends upon following organizational processes that fit our individualistic ways of using our innate brain construction. Sometimes training is needed to guide this process, but the training also must fit our style of thought. We must recognize that there are as many ways to organize as there are individual styles of brain construction. These alternative styles are what this section is about.

The True You will contain its own

workable form of organization—ways that will easily allow you to achieve your goals. Many of the ones covered in this section have been developed by watching what works for creative, analog processing, kinesthenic people.

You will also find continual encouragement to take what pleases you from this suggestion. What doesn't, I encourage you to lay aside, so you avoid further wounding from yet one more approach that doesn't fit you. On occasion, you'll be given suggestions for The Accommodating You so that you can make do until changes in your environment can be accomplished. The Accommodating You will find a path that prevents wounding while getting you where you want to go.

Remember, everyone has a natural pattern of organization within. Let's begin to find yours.

GETTING THE BEST OF CLUTTER

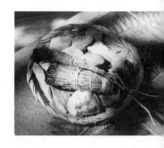

DO YOU STRUGGLE WITH CLUTTER?

Though you have a good-sized office, there's no place for anyone to sit down, or at least not until you clean off a chair. Even when you do clear the papers away from chairs and tabletops, you find they quickly become a repository for more within a short period of time. Even you shake your head in wonderment because you don't remember putting stuff down.

Why this happens:

- When The True You is a creative, hands-on, big picture person, you are likely to have many things that you are doing. These characteristics will lead you to have a lot of "something" that interest you. After all, you may want to make use of the stuff later. Haven't you noticed how many crafts people, inventors, and people who fix things up often have all kinds of things around? For one thing, they keep track of what they have by leaving it in sight. Then, interestingly, they can put what they have saved together in unique ways. That's what creativity is all about.

- You may reflect this same style on your job. Projects needing solutions and goals to be met may all benefit from an artist's style no matter what your business.

- If you've buried things out of sight in a file cabinet, you may not be able to find what you have when you want it. Because you, as a creative, kinesthenic person probably store memories according to how things function, how they feel to you, or by the use you may make of them, you need to be able to openly *see* a reminder that cues a particular memory. One way to do this is to keep "things" out in the open, especially if you stack things according to the projects or interest areas to which they might make a contribution. A file folder covers the content with only a name on a label and is not likely to jog your memory nearly so well.

- If the "stuff" in your life is paper, the task of keeping track of it can be daunting if you are not naturally a one-step-at-a-time person. Unless you stop to read what is on the paper lying on the chair, you won't even know why you're keeping it. Because you can't tell by looking from a distance, you must introduce an extra step into the process of cleaning up the clutter. You must read it. Then you must come up with categories if you are to create a filing system for the paper. That's time consuming at best, daunting at worst. Besides, most of us don't think of this kind of job as creative. Instead, it probably seems boring.

- Perhaps you keep every scrap that crosses your path. But why? If you've been teased or criticized in the past because you couldn't recall facts or the details of a project, you may wish to protect yourself by keeping lots of resources at hand so you can refer back to them, but you rarely will.

What not to do:

Do not get down on yourself for the way your space looks.

What to do:

1. Analyze why your space is the way it is, and then decide what you want to do about it.

2. Check your feelings and see what emotional residue is left over from years of failure to "be organized." Begin the healing of the wounded part of yourself by understanding how The True You works, in this case how you most naturally file resources so you can find them.

3. Remember that you were never trained to organize in ways that could work for you. For example, people with your style of organizing need to sort and file by categories or how things function, not what they're called.

Also you may never have been trained to organize "out in the open" where the things you are working with are visibly available at a glance. With this out-in-the-open approach, you purposely use countertops or floor space to stack the things you're working on. Only finished projects or routine items like forms go in file cabinets.

4. When your feelings get stirred up even thinking about organizing, be understanding and compassionate to both yourself and others in your life who didn't know how to help you. Forgive yourself and them.

5. Start anew with a clean slate to learn to deal with clutter in ways that fit you.

6. Ask yourself, "Do I know where things are in the clutter?"

7. If the answer is yes, consider not changing it. Let this be your private work area.

8. If you need a place to meet other people, create it and don't work in it. It can be a separate room or a screened-off area—just so it's separate. This approach honors The Accommodating You that allows your natural organizational style to interface with the practical world.

9. If you can't find things, analyze why you have so much paper and what you'd like to do about it. Watch out that this isn't what you *think* you *ought* to do about it. Consider having a professional organizer help you. But be sure you choose someone who understands creative, big picture people. The right person will take the time to get to know how you think. He or she will strive to understand your goals. Then the person will help you find a system that fits you—your own system.

Do not let the organizer organize your things. Organizers will tend to do things the way that fits them, not you. Because they will organize according to their own brain construction, you're likely to neither understand the structure, be able to find anything, or maintain whatever system was created.

10. Decide if you want to keep all the paper that comes your way. You probably would do well to simplify your life. To decide whether to do this, ask yourself whether you actually ever use the stuff you've saved previously. It's a myth, for many of us, to think we'll ever recall and track back to the clippings and papers we've saved. Besides, by the time we need them, the item will probably be out of date. Interestingly, as a creative person, you are more than likely to create something new when you need it than find something old that you've saved.

11. Learn a few research skills at your local library or on the Internet and you'll be able to get any up-to-date piece of information you need when you need it.

12. Then clean out everything with a date more than a year old.

What makes this hard to do:

There's a social value placed on neatness with a concomitant criticism of anyone who isn't neat. As a creative, active person, you will have to courageously stand up for the choices you make to work in a way that fits your particular style of brain construction.

Organizing in New Ways

SUBDUING STACKS AND PILES

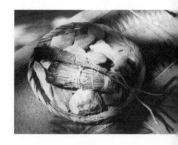

DO YOU HAVE TROUBLE FINDING THE FLOOR IN YOUR HOME OR SPACE FOR YOUR CAR BECAUSE OF THE STACKS AND PILES YOU'VE BUILT?

Sometimes you wonder if your spouse will really divorce you because of the piles of books, magazines, and newspapers you have stacked around your bed, in the corners of your bedroom, and in the garage. You've tried to throw things out, even give them away, but that's very hard for you to do. Even if you manage to do away with a few papers, do you quickly restore the piles to their previous height?

Why this happens:

■ If this scenario looks familiar, you are likely to have a broad vision. You're probably also very active. As a result, you tend to have a lot of things.

■ Ironically, as a person who needs to tangibly see what you have to draw from, you've begun to organize in a way that actually fits you. Your piles and stacks may be considered as resources for what you do: work, education, and entertainment.

- But you've either taken on more than you can do at one time or you are trying to hang onto every interest or idea that crosses your path. Perhaps you feel responsible for everything, i.e., a save-the-world type of person. Or you're fearful that if you let go of anything, ideas, books, or dreams, they will be lost to you forever.

- You may be unsure of your path in life or how to achieve your dreams and are trying to guarantee that you'll find what you are seeking. Every book or magazine reassures you that you'll find your answers.

What not to do:

Do not throw things out indiscriminately or give in to hopeless resignation.

What to do:

1. Make some decisions that will affect your stacks and piles permanently.

2. If the stacks don't bother someone else, it's okay to leave them if you like. You'll need to give yourself permission, however. Check to see if you hear a voice in your head that says stacks are bad and, therefore, it is bad to have them. If you do, tell the voice that you're in control of your life. Say, "Thanks for the suggestions," then do what you want. If the voice is insistent, get tough. Say, "Out of here. I don't need you. I'm in charge." Then get active doing something you want to do, and forget trying to clear out your piles of stuff.

3. If you want to reduce your piles because *you* want to, start with a friend or acquaintance who is willing to help you gain control of your stacks. You will be the one in charge and you will make the decisions. Your helper will be your go-fer.

4. Your first job is to analyze your piles. Both you and your helper can start

with a stack, talking back and forth about what you find. Or your partner can pick up one book or paper at a time, show it to you, and put it where you say it needs to go.

Create a disposable pile and one for items you can't decide about now. You can return to them later. If you ignore this suggestion, you may get bogged down with indecision.

5. Commit to only keep a half dozen or so books near you. Store the rest elsewhere, in a garage or attic, for example. Or give them away to your local library, prison, crisis center, or adult education program. Don't forget you can also have a garage sale.

6. If you decide to keep most of the books you're going through, talk with the person helping you so you come up with categories that allow you to find the items when you want them. Have your partner write these categories down and put labels where you can see them in relation to your stacks. Don't put the labels on the top of the stacks because you'll bury them quickly with other materials. You may wish to consider categories that reflect the content as if you were in a bookstore. You may also find bright colors useful as tags to help you organize according to the subject of an article or book. The color will attract your attention and you are likely to remember the color better than the name of the book or article.

Maybe you have a number of books of varying content that you want to read when you have time. You can store these by order in which you want to read them.

But no matter what order pleases you, use the one that feels best to you. Don't try to be "logical." Your own form of organization needs to prevail. It will if you let it.

7. If you have many interests and ideas and immediately go out and buy books about them as a way to hold

onto them, you can take a new look at what you're doing. Try jotting your idea down on a note card or in your journal rather than keeping a book or article as a reminder—a reminder that takes up space.

8. Consider the notion that just because ideas and interests come into your mind doesn't mean you have to act on every one. Choose one at a time to concentrate on. Send the others back from whence they came so they can be recycled. And remember, if an idea belongs to you, it will come back to your consciousness, nagging at you. You can always choose to focus on it later.

9. If you're searching for your identity in life—who you are or what to do next—your anxiety and fear over not finding it may cause you to grasp at every book or article you can find. Though you can get some answers from these sources, you also can get answers from inside yourself. But you'll need some book-free, quiet thinking and feeling time to do this. Give yourself that time. Later you can savor books without the frenzy attached to your searching.

Also consider spending reading time at the library to satisfy your search for identity rather than bringing the material home.

10. If your stacks bother someone else, remind yourself that living with another person means you must take their wishes into account. You can't arbitrarily expect another person to just accept them, nor does it mean you're a bad person because of your stacks. But mutual respect is a must so you are both satisfied. Reaching a consensus about the stacks is imperative so that both of you feel okay.

If you argue, both wanting your way or wanting control over the situation, you need relationship counseling. Instead, why not spend your time creatively exploring ways to reduce the stacks? If your spouse is

Organizing in New Ways

good at organizing, perhaps you would feel okay about him or her taking the lead to suggest a way to handle them. Give your spouse that power. Do remember, however, that the solution must be one that you are capable of maintaining.

11. Commit to work on one area at a time. (See steps 3–10 as a way to tackle the job.)

     You might want to only work on the stacks that bother your partner the most. Agree to sort those immediately and then take a break. Make a specific agreement to return to the task and set a time for your return.

12. When you finish, treat yourselves to something you both enjoy.

What makes this hard to do:

Spending time organizing or reducing your stacks and piles is a whole lot less pleasurable than acquiring them. But try fully savoring a few books and magazines at a time. Thoroughly read them. Know you'll have time for more when you finish these.

CLEANING THE WHOLE HOUSE

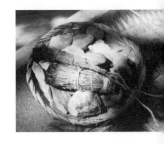

DO YOUR ORGANIZATIONAL SKILLS DEFY YOUR ATTEMPTS TO GET BIG PROJECTS, SUCH AS CLEANING THE HOUSE, DONE?

You have a perfectly good house and would like to see it neat and orderly. But every time you set aside time to clean it, you barely get started before you feel overwhelmed and give up. You get one or two things done and then get distracted. Sometimes you don't get started at all because you have no idea where to start.

Why this happens:

- When you see the housecleaning project as *one big* project, it appears, and is, an *enormous* job.

- Having a brain that sees big pictures means you may not have great skill at seeing the little things that make up the whole picture. So you won't see what needs to be done. Even when you see the little pieces, you may not be able to order the steps to implement them in a way that will systematically get you through your cleaning.

- Trying to use a systematic approach with a house in chaos is hopeless for many people who are not systematic people.

- If you are a creative, inventive person, you may have projects at home—a lot of them. You have a lot of stuff to clean.

- You probably prefer spending time with people or doing exciting things rather than cleaning house.

- The way you were taught you *should* clean house may not work for you.

What not to do:

Do not try to clean your house all at once or use an approach that doesn't fit your style of brain construction.

What to do:

1. First, look at the function of neatness. Ask yourself,

"Is neatness important so I can find things?"

"Do I want to be neat so someone will stop nagging me?"

"Do I want to be neat to please another person or because I think I *should*?"

Get your motivations straight and know you have choices about both the goal of achieving a clean house and how you go about it. Some people find things just fine in cluttered settings. It's your call!

2. Commit to break your housecleaning project into manageable portions and find a style of cleaning that fits you.

3. Think of housecleaning as a *process*, not a one-time job.

4. Set limits on how much time you want to spend and how many rooms

you want to clean at a time and how neat or thoroughly cleaned you want them to be. Let your feelings be your guide. Let's say you have a mobile home, small apartment, cabin, or cottage. It's not very big. You may consider straightening things up throughout. So you set a limit on the depth of cleaning you are going to undertake. Maybe you don't scrub the sinks and tub this week. You just straighten what shows.

If your house is large, you may always need to limit how many rooms or how deeply you want to clean at a given time as well as how much time you want to spend.

5. Next let's look at two styles of cleaning from which to choose. Make your choice based upon how you naturally work.

   Style 1. Here you work with a whole space, moving through as an improvisational dancer might move through the space. You start, for example, at the dining room table where you find something that belongs in the bedroom. On the way to taking the object to the bedroom, you pass something else that belongs in the bedroom. You sweep it up off the floor and proceed on. At the last minute you notice a collection of items that needs to go to the same place. Since there are too many for your already full hands, you bypass them, drop what you have on the bed, and swing back to fill your arms once more with the additional items.

The improvisational dance method takes a lot of steps as you move through your place. But if you like a lot of activity, it may just work for you as you focus on the process rather than the end result of a "most efficient" method. Your energy is expended creatively. As you look back, you may see the wonderful, enjoyable pattern you made as your heart

Organizing in New Ways

and feelings guided you.

Style 2. You choose one small area and clear it completely. This might be one-fourth of a tabletop only. Especially if you are drawn to this style, consider having a friend or family member pick things up for you and ask you what to do with them. You can either tell the helper where to put the items or you may want to have three piles in front of you. One pile is labeled "Throw away." (Consider having a garbage bag on hand in that spot.) The second pile might be labeled, "I can't live without this." And the third pile is called, "I don't know."

You may only get a small number of things into the piles the first day, but that is progress. Then commit to another time to work with your helper to put away the things you can't live without. As for the "I don't know" pile, put it away for six months in a storage place and don't worry about it. At the end of the storage period, sort it into three piles once more. Each time you do this, your pile will dwindle in size until it disappears.

6. If during your big project cleaning you become overwhelmed, you may be trying to do too much or for too long. Break the amount of work you do into smaller bits.

7. Once you've cleared away some space, commit to bringing less stuff into your house. Do not buy or bring anything home until you've used up or passed on something.

8. As for having a place to put what you have, make choices that appeal to you. If "out of sight, out of mind" rules your organizational world, remember that open shelves and tabletops are free for storing and filing things you use frequently.

9. Have special, out-of-the-way places

for creative, inventive projects—places where you can leave unfinished work out in the open. Then only clean up *after* you finish a project, but only if you want to. If you leave things out, be sure they're in a place that's yours and not where everyone else in the house has to look at them.

10. If you like to spend time with people, relate clean-up time to having someone over—which then becomes your motivation. Also consider having someone over while you work, even if that person only talks to you.

11. Culturally, the importance of house-cleaning varies. Some folks rank it very high on their list of "musts." Others place less value on it. Some people even place neatness fairly far down on their priority list.

Decide how much you value neatness. Talk with the people with whom you live and find ways to meet everyone's needs. It's not a matter of right or wrong, but purposeful choice. Be sure to take yourself into consideration as well as others.

What makes this hard to do:

It takes time to discover a system that works for you. And finding the right one is complex. So first work on your motives. Then find the style you wish to follow and practice it, training yourself over time.

Organizing in New Ways

KEEPING TRACK OF PERSONAL FINANCES

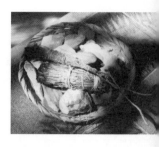

DO YOU FIND YOU'RE CONTINUALLY HAVING TROUBLE KEEPING UP WITH BILLS AND FINANCIAL INFORMATION?

Keeping track of bills, receipts, and bank statements is ruining your life. You can't find the bills you need to pay. You don't have any idea where the receipt is to return something to the store. And worst of all, you have no idea where to find what you need to file your income tax, much less what to do about the other years you haven't filed even though you meant to. You feel hopeless.

Why this happens:

■ Keeping bills and receipts is a very linear, detailed job—one that does not use the skills that may make up your strengths. If you are a big picture person who sees the overview of situations and automatically pays attention to how things function or are used, you may be able to recall a picture of when and why you generated the bills and receipts, but not actually *find* them. The individual bits of paper are not a part of your perceptual world.

■ Storing bits of paper means you need to find a system that will work for you. Most organizational systems are not designed for creative, global processors of information who respond to colors and patterns and need lots of activity to implement any job.

■ When you are the type of person who feels deeply and would rather be in relationships than tinker with numbers and details, you will have trouble keeping track of your personal finances. That's the down side of the way The True You experiences the world, requiring you to find ways to build The Accommodating You who can keep up with required personal economic matters.

■ If you haven't found a system that does work for you, you are likely to feel wounded by expectations beyond your control. It doesn't take long until pure chaos takes over and you have absolutely no idea where or how to start. Panic and avoidance are the likely result.

■ finally, shame over being out of control is likely to keep you immobilized, as secondary wounding deepens your original hurt. The Wounded You takes over, leaving little or no capability to do the task.

What not to do:

Don't do "nothing." But also, don't beat up on yourself.

What to do:

1. Ask for help. Bring your situation out into the open and find people who can help you immediately. Later, when this crisis is over, you can work on discovering an organizational system that fits you, so you never again have to become desperate.

2. Come face to face with the reality of

your situation, admitting that you're out of control with a task that The Accommodating You must find a solution to while avoiding further wounding.

3. Bite the bullet. Cast shame aside. Assuming you aren't trying to avoid payment, you have nothing to be ashamed of. You must get past the immobilizing effects of what belongs to your past. Forgive yourself and get on with getting the job done.

4. If you once had a system that worked for you, at least some of the time—one that did not create an inordinate amount of stress—recall when and why you stopped using it. Sometimes major life stresses get us off track: divorce, health problems, moving.

5. If this happened, dust off the system. Recall how it worked.

6. You may have found that having a special place to put your bills and receipts helps you become habituated to placing them there so they don't get lost. Organizing using colored folders may help you keep track of your financial things because of a tendency to be drawn to color, or maybe all your receipts get put in a basket until you decide to sort them. You may want to stack financial matters that need telephone intervention next to your phone. Computer-related projects go next to your computer. Maybe you've had a table or a place on the floor that you marked off for a specific project, such as collecting what you need to take to the accountant for your income tax. You've probably also noticed that it is only wise to put papers away, out of sight, *after* you've finished working on them.

7. Perhaps you learned to make lists. There, too, color coding probably proved useful.

8. Commit to use again whatever you liked about your old system.

9. Ask someone to help you catch up using the old system. Being a "people person," you will likely respond to this approach.

10. Set small, achievable goals and congratulate yourself every time you reach one. For example, if you are trying to get your income tax papers (receipts and ledgers) together, start sorting what lays on the tabletop in one room. Have a file folder or box to put the papers in to take to your accountant. If you need to, take one batch at a time so you get the papers out of your house as soon as possible.

11. If you have no history with a system that worked for you, it's time to find one. find a system or person who can help you develop a system that will work for you. If a person is helping you, that person must be able to *read* you and your reactions to every suggestion, not bring in a premade system and expect you to fit into it.

Any organizational system only fits a segment of the population. If you're not drawn to a system, don't pressure yourself to continue.

12. Be willing to try several approaches during your period of investigation.

13. Seriously consider permanently hiring or making a trade with someone to manage the personal paperwork in your life.

14. This may be a painful time, but once you're caught up, you can see you don't get in this mess again. Later, if you get off track, you can jump back on right away using the system you like best.

What makes this hard to do:

Your style of brain construction can make dealing with your personal

Organizing in New Ways

finances next to impossible. The feelings of shame and guilt that result tend to make you hide from it. Being overwhelmed keeps you from making headway in dealing with it. Not knowing where to start gets in the way.

The problem is that the IRS and bill collectors won't go away. So face the music sooner rather than later. You may not be talented in handling paperwork, but you are not a bad person because you're having trouble. Ask for help to accommodate to a job that doesn't fit the way you're made.

MANAGING PAPER AT WORK

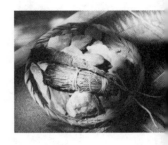

DO YOU DO WONDERFULLY ON YOUR JOB EXCEPT FOR THE PAPERWORK?

You are skillful at all aspects of your job except keeping track of what you've accomplished. You are a skilled people-person who is expressive and creative, but you sure have trouble keeping up with your paperwork. You're not alone. You probably know someone who's very talented and may be self-employed who has the same problem you do. Tracking expenditures, sales, profits, time, mileage, and even income is beyond both of you.

Why this happens:

- In essence, you are being called upon to do two or more totally different jobs under the label of one.

- Each job requires the use of different areas of your brain. The area that manages accounting and keeps track of details is a different area than the part that makes you so talented and skillful in the important areas of your job—the ones you like.

- Rarely, if ever, are people equally good at both types of skills.

What not to do:

Do not expect yourself to necessarily be good at everything on the job. But don't avoid the parts that are hard. They will catch up with you sooner or later.

What to do:

1. Learn ways to manage paperwork that fit your brainstyle.

2. Make a list either mentally or on paper of what you do and don't do well on your job.

3. Notice similarities between the items in each list.

4. If you can, partner with someone on the job to do the tasks that are hard for you. Make a trade to do something that is hard for the other person. You might exchange speaking in front of a group for bookkeeping, for example.

5. If you can't find someone with whom to make a trade, talk to your boss about having someone keep track of your clerical work. Point out that you'll bring in more business or create more product with the help you receive. The clerical help will end up paying for itself.

6. If you have to do the job yourself, go easy on yourself so you don't waste energy on self-blame.

7. Ask yourself whether you are the kind of person who does better doing a little bit of something hard and then taking a break. If so, you probably want to deal with your paperwork daily or even after every sale or accomplishment.

8. Set yourself up in an environment that fits you. Maybe you love the out-of-doors, so you feel better if

you do your clerical work outside. Or maybe you like to have music playing or someone to keep you company while you do the work that comes with difficulty.

9. For certain, reward yourself when you're done. Treat yourself to something you like: a tennis game, your favorite food, or a movie, whatever pleases you.

10. If you prefer to do your organizational work all at once, then do it that way. Work on your accounts weekly or file monthly. Do what feels best.

11. Give yourself permission to be responsible in your own way.

12. Never hesitate to ask for help.

What makes this hard to do:

Although people who are usually good at clerical work are not expected to be creative or particularly expressive or mechanical, everyone is expected to be able to do clerical work. You are not allowed to say, "I'm not talented at clerical work," whereas others may say, "I'm not creative, musically, artistically, or mechanically."

WRITING A REPORT

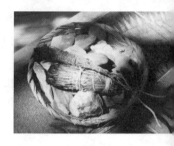

DO YOU SPEND WAY TOO MUCH TIME ORGANIZING A REPORT AND STILL NOT DO A VERY GOOD JOB?

You are writing a report. Though you produce this kind of document regularly, you always spend a very long time trying to get it organized. You try to write an outline ahead of time, but you don't seem to be able to make that work for you. And you're pretty sure your end result isn't very good. You dread writing it.

Why this happens:

■ As someone who *feels* your way through a writing task, or any project for that matter, you are not likely to be able to begin at the beginning. Neither do you think or write in little steps. Instead, when you begin a task such as this, you probably have the information for the report churning around in your mind with no beginning, middle, or end in sight.

■ Yet a paper or any big project requires a lot of steps in order to put it together. Although you may be able to see the finished goal in all its entirety, that does not mean you'll be able to know the steps that lead to that goal.

■ Having a sense of what you want to accomplish for the project may be what invigorates you, not taking the steps to accomplish it.

■ You might even be better able to speak the report than write it.

What not to do:

Do not give up because you feel you'll never be able to produce a worthwhile report.

What to do:

1. Learn to break the project up into small sections that you can order in a way that will allow you to finish. This does not necessarily mean you start at the beginning.

2. Be clear about whom the report is being written for, what the goal of the report is, when it is to be done, and whether you'll need to do the same kind of report (project) repeatedly. These are the parameters that will help you find a structure for the report.

3. Brainstorm. Do this alone, with someone else, or even in a group. On a piece of paper or blackboard, write down as many components of the report as you can. Anything you think of that's related to the report gets written at this time. This could include introduction, background, conclusions, summary, explanation of new events since the last report, effects of the new events, key players, and so on.

   Use single words or short phrases. Draw pictures. Do not necessarily put the ideas down in a list, though that's okay. Remember, there really are no rules to brainstorming.

Organizing in New Ways

Another way to begin organizing your report is to put each idea related to the project down on a card and lay the cards on the floor or all over a table.

4. When you can't think of anything else, take a deep breath and a break.

5. When you're ready to go to work again, step back from the words you've accumulated. This way you can scan them all together. You may instantly see items that go together, even the categories in which to fit them. You'll *feel* what goes together. This way of approaching organization fits your brainstyle.

   You may wish to read the words aloud. Notice which subjects draw your attention repeatedly. Perhaps you keep noticing two words together. It could mean that the two subjects belong together in the report.

   You may start with twenty-five items. Then divide these twenty-five into several groups, making large

categories. You're beginning to create clusters. One cluster will seem to precede another cluster as the paper starts to take shape.

6. Now decide which section of the paper to work on next. Again, you do not necessarily have to start at the beginning. Let your feelings guide you.

7. You may find it more effective to work on the whole project a little at a time rather than working on one section and honing it to completion before turning to the next section.

   A big picture person makes several run-throughs of the whole report—one run for content, one to be sure the sections are connected the way you want them, another for editing, and so on.

8. When you are done, and maybe a time or two during the writing, let the report set for a time. When you

go back, you'll more clearly see what you want to change.

9. If you have to write this same or a similar document in the future, outline the paper *after* it is finished. Then you can use that same outline the next time. You'll be able to use it because you created it in your own way in the first place.

10. If you really feel lost, don't hesitate to ask someone to help you. You could contact an editor to edit your work. You can hire or make a trade with someone to create an outline for you.

    Choose someone you like and someone who likes you and respects your work. This way you are more likely to be on the same wavelength. And that person is more likely to be able to help you while honoring your style and approach. You and your skills and talents will be respected.

What makes this hard to do:

Your worst enemy may be your feelings. Feeling overwhelmed with no idea of where to start can block your progress. Thinking you *ought* to start at the beginning and work sequentially through to the end may stall your progress.

Be sure to breathe and use your inner feelings to see what you're drawn to do, one step at a time, no matter what your order of writing.

PUTTING OFF STARTING THINGS

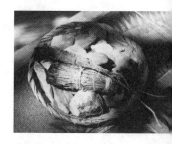

DO YOU PROCRASTINATE STARTING PROJECTS?

You have a report to write. It's due on Friday. Every month, you promise yourself you'll start it earlier, but you never really get around to working on it until Wednesday afternoon or Thursday. You don't mind doing it. And you always get it done even if you have to stay up late to finish it.

A lot of people have made fun of you and even question you about not starting things earlier. You were the same way in school. Even though you actually do a quality job, you are concerned that you may need to change. But you don't know how because you've tried many times and never succeeded.

Why this happens:

- All your life you've probably been told you *should* begin things early. You feel that it's wrong to put off getting going. You've been labeled a *procrastinator* and that's *not* a good thing to be. You probably believe it means there's something *wrong* with you. But the reason you have the pattern of production you have is because of your style of brain construction.

- Some people naturally work better when they wait until a deadline is due. Then their creative juices mobilize all at once for the creative activity.

- This is especially true of people who see the big picture. Some people work on a project in their mind, even out of their conscious awareness, working out the details, and then discovering that the project comes out in one whole unit.

- We all have our own rhythm for working and doing. Many spontaneous, creative people get an assignment, check out the parameters of it, and then tuck the assignment in the back of their minds. Two or three or more days later, they consider the assignment again, rechecking its parameters: the intended audience,

its purpose, and its length. Then they begin writing and the whole thing comes out all at once. Often little rearranging is needed. All that's left is a bit of editing and the job is done. This is simply another style of approaching a project from the more typical step-by-step approach.

- There is a belief that early planning followed by doing a little bit on the project at regular intervals is preferable to taking the approach that works best for big picture people. But it's a belief that only fits some styles of brain construction, not all.

What not to do:

Do not get down on yourself because you put things off to the last minute. Do not try to fit a production schedule that's not made for your particular style of brain construction.

Organizing in New Ways

What to do:

1. Be sure you are willing to do the project at hand.

2. Give yourself permission to work on any project in your own way in your own time.

3. As you are learning of the project, be certain you understand the parameters of the assignment. Ask yourself the following questions.

    "Who am I doing the project for?"

    "What do I need to get across in it?"

    "How long does it need to be?"

    "How long do I estimate it will take me to do it if I do it all at once?"

4. Look at a month-at-a-glance calendar and mark when the project is due. Subtract one day for miscellaneous problems like a failed printer cartridge. Next, ask yourself how long you'd like to spend working on the actual construction of the whole project. Subtract this time. Now you'll know when you'll probably need to begin the actual production. You'll check this estimate with your feelings later.

5. Are there any special preparations you need to make, special materials to be ordered, people to interview, or research to do? Mark on your calendar when you want to accomplish these tasks, not when you think you *should* do them.

6. Now put the project in the back of your mind. Your brain will be working on the formulation of it whether you're consciously thinking about the project or purposely doing anything about it.

7. Do the tasks you've assigned yourself at the assigned times, but don't push yourself to begin the actual writing

or production until you *feel* it's time to start. Compare the time you estimated earlier with your current feeling of whether it is the *right* time for you to begin. Hopefully they'll match. If not, listen carefully to your feeling *and* think about the discrepancy, then come to a consensus.

8. Finally, when the time comes to begin work, review the parameters, who, what, and how. (This is a very important part of the plan.) Close your eyes, take a deep breath, and ask your creative self to begin the process. Within seconds, a picture, word, or thought will jump into your mind. With that, you're off and running.

9. Capture whatever comes to you, and you'll find you've already started.

10. Let whatever follows flow through you. In all probability, the whole thing will come out at once with little or no cutting and pasting nec-

essary. You may be surprised at how well the pieces fit together as they flow out of you in order.

11. When you're criticized for your style, simply tell people you have the situation under control and you'll take responsibility for completing the project in a timely manner. When you begin working this new way, you may need to practice a little to adjust your timing. That's to be expected. Just don't throw out this new way of doing your work because your initial timing needs some adjusting. You'll be fine before long.

What makes this hard to do:

Changing a belief about yourself and the way in which you work is hard. You'll have to convince yourself that it's okay to do assignments in your own way.

Organizing in New Ways

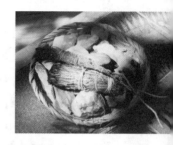

TALKING OFF TRACK

DO YOU GET OFF TRACK WHEN YOU ARE TALKING?

You are giving a talk and you start to give an example or tell a story that describes a point you are trying to make. The next thing you know, you can't remember what you were saying before you took the mental side trip.

Why this happens:

- As a person whose brain focuses on the patterns, interconnections, and relationships between things more than on specific bits of information, you are likely to drift away from one thought to a complex of thoughts. That's just how you are made.

- The True You is a big picture person who tends to tell stories and describe whole scenes to make your point when you're speaking. Think of yourself as heading down a straight path toward a goal. You are describing what you see to others. You see something to the side of the path that will enrich your description, perhaps even make it more understandable. You decide to share what you see.

You get off the main track, creating a side trip.

- You will also tend to get totally immersed in what you're doing. This immersion temporarily makes you forget what you were saying earlier while you were on the main path.

- You are also likely to experience shame over "losing your train of thought." Then, feeling shame, you are likely to become further distracted as you pay attention to your feelings.

What not to do:

Do not let yourself feel helplessly lost from your original path.

What to do:

1. Learn to anchor your initial thought while enriching your speaking with side trips.

2. Concentrate on identifying the desire to add something to whatever you're talking about.

3. Make a purposeful decision to take the side trip.

4. Verbalize that decision to the person you're speaking to or to someone in your audience. This is what anchoring is. You anchor the point at which you get off your path to the person.

5. Note where you are placing your anchor with a gesture, such as pointing your finger downward as if you were casting an anchor into the water. Hold your hand in that position all the time you are telling the example. Or you may want to touch another's arm, probably the person you're talking to, holding that position until you are finished with the example.

6. When talking to a group, you can ask someone in the audience to

remember where you leave the path. Ironically, having asked, you'll probably remember yourself.

7. When you are ready to return to the main theme of your talking, simply look in the direction of the anchor, i.e., your pointed finger or the person you anchored to. Then take up where you left off. Amazingly, you *will* remember where you left off.

What makes this hard to do:

Embarrassment and fear that you won't be able to overcome getting off track may make it hard for you to change. Perhaps you think you shouldn't need to do anything to stay on track. These fears often make us feel helpless to change our situation. Just remember, you are not helpless.

GETTING PLACES ON TIME

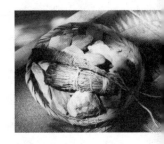

DO YOU RUN THE RISK OF NOT GETTING IMPORTANT PLACES ON TIME?

The idea of missing a scheduled airplane flight fills you with anxiety, but your fear doesn't seem to do much for getting you to the airport on time. Last time, you not only came close to missing your flight but also jeopardized your colleague's getting there on time. Repeatedly, you've promised yourself you'll do better, but you keep failing.

Why this happens:

- Intending to leave early enough to get somewhere on time does not mean you know how to do it.

- Figuring out the amount of time you need to accomplish a task can be very difficult for those people with a large number of analog processing attributes. "Telling time" by a clock, especially a digital clock, and "keeping time" are linear activities involving *unnatural* measurements such as minutes and hours. This is in opposition to telling time by using the natural rhythms of nature, such as watching the sun or using your own body rhythms.

■ You may be using the wrong type of clock for your brain construction.

■ If you are untrained to be in touch with your natural environment, you may think you have more time than you actually do to get somewhere. Let's say you round off a target number to the nearest half or quarter hour. For example, if your plane leaves at 6:47 P.M., you may think of it as 7 P.M. But in so doing, you've lost thirteen minutes. Lost minutes accumulate.

■ Often the suggestion is made to simply add fifteen or thirty minutes to the time you would normally leave to go somewhere. Even when applied to situations involving the same schedule repeatedly, it doesn't work. People with this problem know they've added the time and come up with all kinds of ways to fill in that additional time. Thus you end up leaving later than ever.

■ Being an active person, you tend to get involved in lots of activities at the same time, including doing things that have nothing to do with getting to your destination on time.

What not to do:

Do not ignore the problem, compounding your guilt and jeopardizing your job or a relationship.

What to do:

1. Believe that you can get your timing under control in a way that will work for your natural self.

2. Commit to work on your time management.

3. Use an analog clock. Though less precise, it gives you a better sense of the time. You can look quickly at the

clock and sense whether you're close to the hour (12), just past the quarter hour (3), midway to the half hour (6), or considerably past the three-quarter hour (9). These estimates will give you a clear feeling for what time it is. Work with these quarter-hour segments, rounding up to the top end of the fifteen minutes rather than the lower number.

4. To get to a destination such as an airport on time, you must break the time span needed to get there into segments. Once you've figured out how much time you need to spend in preparation and travel to the destination, you will automatically and easily be able to know when to leave in the future. Then you'll have the structure you need for all your trips to that destination.

5. To take a trip to the airport as an example, work backwards to figure your timetable. Ask yourself some questions.

"How much ahead of time do I need to arrive at the gate?" Answer: One hour.

"How long will it take me to park and get to the terminal?" Answer: Thirty minutes. Add another thirty minutes if it's the time of day when spaces are scarce or it's a holiday.

"How long will it take me to drive to the airport?" Answer: Forty-five minutes. Add thirty minutes if you are driving during rush hour.

"How long will it take me to do errands between my house and the airport?" This includes getting gas, dropping off dry cleaning, etc. Answer: Fifteen minutes.

6. You now have the time you need between leaving your residence or office and arriving at your destination. In this case it's two and a half hours.

7. Next figure how much time it takes to get ready to leave your house.

Wake up: Fifteen minutes.

Shower/bath: Fifteen minutes.

Shave/make-up: Fifteen minutes.

Dress: Fifteen minutes.

Cook and eat: Fifteen minutes.

Feed pets: Fifteen minutes.

Deal with kids: Thirty minutes.

Close house: Fifteen minutes.

You may wish to pack the night before unless you're leaving late in the day.

8. As you figure your timing, remember to round off upward every amount you require to the nearest fifteen-minute segment (12, 3, 6, 9).

9. Find the total time you need. Perhaps you find you need two and a half hours between the time you leave your house and get to the airport. And you find you need two hours and fifteen minutes from the time you get up until you leave home.

10. Note what time your plane leaves. Round this off to the half hour. (If your plane leaves at 8:37, figure it will leave at 8:30.)

11. If it takes you two and a half hours to get to the airport, you must leave your office or house at 6:00 A.M. If it takes you two hours and fifteen minutes between the time you get up and the time you leave your house, you'll get up at 3:45. No if, ands, or buts. You get up then.

12. When you book your flight, *immediately* calculate your timing. Or if the thought of doing this overwhelms you, ask someone else to do it. Then leave at the time you've figured.

13. Post the time in your calendar book and put up a sticky note on the door. And leave at that time. If you're only half dressed or don't have your make-up on, leave anyway. That will encourage you to be timely in the future. Besides, you can put on your make-up at your destination because you'll have time.

14. It may take you a flight or two to work the bugs out of your timing. While this is happening, you may not want to take on the responsibility for a second person. Either let your colleague pick you up (and remember, go as you are rather than keep the person waiting), or tell that person to go separately until you get your timing under control.

15. If you characteristically keep your spouse or coworker waiting, tell him or her to go on ahead. If you're not ready, under no circumstances should that person wait for you.

16. Take something to read in case you get to your destination early.

What makes this hard to do:

The biggest problem comes when someone takes responsibility for your timing while you are learning. You must be certain that no one is waiting on you. That person is short-changing you, robbing you of your ability to learn to be responsible. You may have to be very emphatic with someone who unwittingly sabotages your progress this way.

Another hindrance comes from someone nagging you to "get going." The natural reaction is to move even slower in opposition to the nagging. Simply say, "You're not helping. I'd appreciate your backing off. I'll take care of things."

What also makes time management hard is that you are dealing with a habit that may be long standing, and habits are always hard to break. But you can do it.

Organizing in New Ways

REFUELING YOUR ENERGY

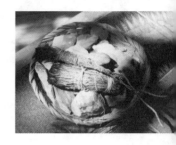

DO YOU HAVE TROUBLE ORGANIZING YOUR EATING AND SLEEPING HABITS?

Okay, so you skip breakfast most days. Then you often grab a candy bar or two during the day and keep going with lots and lots of coffee or diet drinks loaded with caffeine. It takes too much time to find healthy food and too much organization to eat regularly.

And, yes, your sleep habits aren't much better. It's just that you have a hard time getting to sleep at night and an even harder time getting up. You seem to be tired all the time.

No two days in your life are the same. You seem healthy enough now but . . . you wonder whether you'll pay later for such sloppy habits.

Why this happens:

- As a baby, you may have had trouble settling into a *regular* schedule. Sensitive infants can have a tough time settling into the world of booming, buzzing, clattering confusion that prevails in most households, especially those with energetic, multitasking parents.

- Individuals have their own internal time clocks. Some of us are day people and others come alive at night. Though it is possible for each type to participate in the other's world, it's not easy. But today's world strongly favors day people, which puts a great burden on those who do well at night.

- If you have a lot of sensitivity to stimuli that distract you from your work, you may prefer nighttime for working because it is quiet. You're less likely to be interrupted.

- When you don't naturally fit the demands of the timetable that defines your life, you are likely to need energy boosters to keep going, such as coffee and chocolate.

- Eating regularly means you must make the time to do that, which also means you will be on a regular schedule. But if you are a "go with the flow" type of person, you probably don't live on a regular schedule and don't much want to. That means you "keep going" using whatever you can get your hands on to provide you with energy.

- Nutritious meals are not easily available on fast food row. It takes planning to get fresh produce and meats in a timely manner. It takes time to prepare interesting nutritious meals. If your time is limited and you're not a natural cook, the whole business of meal production may seem too complicated. Besides, you may rarely be home to accomplish it.

What not to do:

Do not give up on the idea of eating nutritiously and getting satisfactory sleep.

What to do:

1. Do find a natural eating and sleeping schedule that fits you.

Organizing in New Ways

2. Go on a campaign to find nutritious but easy to obtain foods that you like.

3. Spend the next month seeking out a way to get these foods easily so that you don't have to make an *effort* to eat regularly and nutritiously. Not every eating style or type of diet is good for all people. You'll need to experiment a bit to find what you need. Do not listen to the advertisements that tout a special diet for everyone.

    If you're the kind of person who likes to *study* things in depth, systematically check out different kinds of foods that you like and stick to them, making sure that you have a balance of protein foods, fresh greens and vegetables, fruits, and some treats. Add milk products if your body tolerates them.

4. Now decide if you want to eat out or at home most of the time. If you prefer to eat out, find places that will cater to your needs. You'd be surprised how adaptive most cooks and chefs are these days. Let them know what you want. You can also take your food to go if you want to eat it on the run. You can simulate fast food expedience by calling ahead, and you won't have to wait. Or you might even have your food delivered.

5. You can get home cooking if you make a trade with someone, a partner, friend, or neighbor, who is willing to cook for you. In exchange you can trade anything from baby sitting to carpentry repair or lawn mowing.

6. If you don't want to mess with food every day, make enough to feed you for a week. Maybe you cook two chickens, several pounds of meat (ribs, ground or sliced meat) and fish, a big batch of rice, and a batch of potatoes. You can even make a huge salad, storing it without dressing.

    Store each type of food separately,

freezing part of it in individual containers. Also keep frozen or canned vegetables on hand all the time. When you're preparing to leave for the day (or night), put some of a variety of the foods in a container—one that you can put in a microwave works well. If you want, you can sprinkle cheese on the top. Heat it until it is very hot. Seal it and off you go. Or you can wait to heat it at the workplace if a microwave is available. You can even eat it at room temperature. An insulated picnic basket will get you through the summer months.

7. At work you can keep a bottle of salad dressing and some taste enhancers such as nuts, seeds, dried fruit, seasonings, grated cheese, and other "goodies." This will change the taste of the food. But only add this step if it appeals to you. If it adds stress, forget it.

8. Stock up on healthy snack food that you leave in your vehicle or desk. Dried foods, jerky, nuts and fruits, and vegetables all make wonderful pick-me-ups.

9. It really doesn't much matter what you eat or how you combine it if you eat a balanced diet and it's fresh, additive-free food that is moderately low in processed sugar and fats. Watch out for advertising where sugar is substituted for fat or a synthetic additive is substituted for sugar and the label says "Nutritious" or "Healthy." A balance of food types, freshness, naturalness, and foods that fit your system and the season are the key to healthy living.

10. As for sleep, you would do well to look closely at your own natural rhythms. Everyone has them. Working with them rather than against them is a good idea. There are programs that attempt to retrain people to fit the standard 8 to 5 daytime schedule. But does it make

sense to you to tamper with nature unless absolutely necessary? It tends to stress your system.

11. Adults have more flexibility than children, who generally must be in school during certain hours. More and more parents are homeschooling, in part because the school schedule can be a major disruption of some children's natural sleep rhythms and interferes with their learning as well as their own well-being. For adults, there is a whole world of night work. It's a world unto itself. If you are a natural night owl, explore it. Or consider self-employment of a kind that lends itself to a flexible sleep/wake cycle.

12. Experiment with split shifts and naps of varying lengths. Some folks can take a five-minute nap and keep going for hours. Others need lengthy periods of sleep to recuperate.

13. Pay no attention to anyone who says you should sleep a particular number of hours a night. This, too, is extremely variable, person to person. If you only need to sleep a few hours a night, so be it. Tell the person, "Thank you for your concern, but I'm in charge of my sleeping." Then, don't talk about your sleep habits.

14. Check to see that you do get enough sleep, however, to be responsible with your commitments. If you have a class at 8 A.M. and like to stay up late, you may need to be sure you get a midday nap so you can meet your 8 A.M. obligation. Then as soon as you can, create a schedule that fits you better.

What makes this hard to do:

Believing that there is a *right* time and way to sleep and eat presses you into a pattern that is *wrong* for you. You must counteract this belief by standing up for what The True You naturally responds to. Discover the means that fit you.

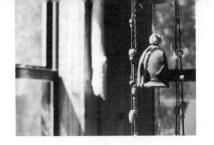

PART TWO

Following Through to Success

We can learn to gather information from all parts of ourselves, not just our heads.

LINDA JEAN SHEPHERD, PH.D.

1993

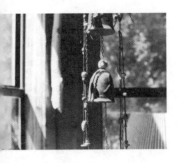

Practical, everyday life teaches us to keep our eye on our goal, if we are to succeed. Yet, do we not often feel we've failed to achieve our goals in a timely manner, getting off track or not traveling in the straight line that we've been taught is the way to achieve outcomes?

Brainstyle not only shapes the nature of the goals that interest us but the manner in which we strive toward them. For some of us, the shortest, fastest, straight-line approach may work well. But for many others of us, providing a broader range of experience as we travel to the goal not only better fits our innate brain-style but yields the kind of end product we desire.

This section urges The True You to become sensitive to alternative ways to achieve the goals you desire. Guidelines to avoid getting and staying off track because of the particular way in which you do things will help The Accommodating You avoid stress and loss. Best of all, new hope for successful follow-through to goals you previously thought were out of reach will allow you to enjoy the success of accomplishment.

MAKING A BIG PURCHASE

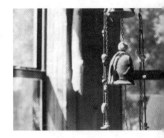

DO YOU FEEL YOU'RE *SUPPOSED* TO DO RESEARCH BEFORE MAKING A BIG PURCHASE?

Last week you and your wife made a decision that the time had come when it only makes sense to buy a house. Your kids are approaching school age, and you and she have enough income to take this step. You felt excited and immediately began to drive through neighborhoods so you could get a *feel* for where you'd like to live. You thought you might even see a house that you'd really like.

Yesterday you and your wife sat down to talk some more. As you compared notes, you discovered to your amazement that your wife had not gone out to look at a single house. Instead, she had a piece of paper with a list of attributes she felt were important when buying a house. She'd checked to see what different schools' test scores were last year. She talked to friends and acquaintances about safe neighborhoods. She scanned market values and had what seemed like a whole encyclopedia of facts about areas in which to live that would be convenient for both of you to get to work. She even knew where the shopping centers were and an estimate of the time it would take to get to the grocery store from various neighborhoods. She had plans for how much you could afford as a down payment and how much your mortgage payments and insurance would cost.

When it was your turn to share what you'd done, all you could say was, "Well, I liked such and such a neighborhood. And there is a wonderful-looking house for sale on First Street. I love the way it looks."

Immediately your wife, trying to be supportive, said, "What's the asking price for the house on First Street? What school district is it in? How much equity does the owner have in the house?"

You couldn't answer any of her questions. You just *liked* the house. You had already thought of some of the questions your wife asked, but mostly you wanted to see if your wife liked it, too, before you went any further. Why even consider such questions if she didn't like a house?

You realize how differently you each approached the prospect of buying a house. You are a little worried that maybe you'll end up with a house that is sensible but won't be something *wonderful.* On the other hand, you feel embarrassed that you hadn't approached this project *sensibly,* like your wife.

Why this happens:

- Opposites attract. Though you know this, you may not have thought about brainstyle differences as opposites attracting. Only now are you beginning to realize the profound effect of brainstyle on each and every aspect of your relationship.

- You have an approach to life that is shaped primarily by your feelings. The part of your brain that processes feelings is strong. You experience the styles and tones of things and are probably quite creative by nature. You are likely to relate to the patterns created by what you see and the relationships between what you see and what is around it. For example, you'll notice how the house looks in relation to the land upon which it sits. You'll notice the shape of the house in silhouette against the sky, how close it is to other houses, to foliage, etc. You may have noted whether you'll be able to see the sunrise or sunset from the porch. This is what is important to you.

In contrast, your wife may process little of this information. Instead, she will think about the details involved in buying the house, the specifics of everyday travel, the so-called practical aspects. She may be concerned about the local school district's test scores while you may be concerned with whether there are trees for climbing and room for running and exploring. It's not that each of you isn't concerned about all of these things. Rather, it's what you think about and look for first. You might call it the "lead system" of The True You.

■ If you feel embarrassed, it's because the culture in which you live teaches that practical details are more important than feelings and aesthetics.

What not to do:

Do not feel bad *or* superior about the way in which you go about making a decision.

What to do:

1. Do combine your approaches, creating a team approach to making a big purchase.

2. When you sit down together, take turns leading the discussion. When your partner leads it, they can take charge of listing all the particulars that need to be considered from the vantage point that comes easily for them.

3. Next they can interview you in rela-

Following Through to Success
_____

tion to the items they've listed. That way both of you have input into that aspect of the project.

4. It's your turn next. This time you talk about what you want in a house: feeling, tone, style, color, and so on. Also note what you don't want. You are not likely to create a list. Instead you will probably see pictures in your mind or recall memories of houses you've liked and will paint a picture of these to your partner.

5. Next draw out your partner's preferences. Dialogue. See what they like. It's important to let them talk freely even if they come up with some things you dislike. If they say that a style or a feeling doesn't matter because you have to go with a house that's well built regardless of style, simply pose the situation where you have two houses, both of which are equal except for style. Ask your partner which they would prefer.

6. When you both have finished, make a list of issues and items that are essential for each of you. You don't have to agree. All it takes is one person who feels adamantly about a point to get it on the list. This is a kind of "I can't/won't live with/without this" list.

7. Under no conditions put down the other person or that person's suggestions. Also do not argue about something that's a "have to" for one of you. Join forces to find a house that has the basics you each want.

8. Next look at what you'd like but can live without.

9. Continue looking at houses either separately or together.

10. Meet regularly to compare notes and congratulate one another for the perspective you each contribute.

11. When you come to an aspect that one of you likes and one doesn't, consider how important it is. Brainstorm how you can create a solution for the one who isn't pleased. For example, if a front porch is a crucial item for one of you and the house in question doesn't have one, could it be added on? What would it take? That might just do the trick.

12. Realize that this decision is not a forever decision. You may find your dream home now. Or you may have to buy two or more houses before you find the home of your dreams.

You may even have to build it one day. But for now, know you've used teamwork to get started as home-owners.

What makes this hard to do:

Many decisions can be very emotional activities, especially when two people have markedly different styles of brain construction. Even people who love each other often may have distinctly different preferences. It will take mutual caring, understanding, and creativity to bridge the gap that opens between the way you each go about making big decisions.

Following Through to Success

FAILING TO FOLLOW THROUGH

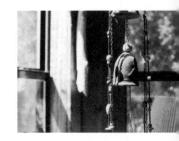

DO YOU FEEL THAT YOU FAIL TO FOLLOW THROUGH ON CHORES?

You plan to do home repair chores on your day off, but by late afternoon you've failed to achieve most of your goal. You have had several good conversations with friends, found some interesting new information about your hobby, and taken a much needed physical break as you played ball with your kids. But you didn't get your chores done.

Why this happens:

■ The most common reason for lack of follow-through is that you have committed to do something you "should" do, not something you want to do.

■ You may be a person who has a lot of interest in relationships—more interest in people than in spending time doing *things*, especially on your day off.

■ You may live in the here and now,

flowing through your day one moment at a time with your focus on the present rather than on some future goal, especially on your day off. As a result, you lose contact with your goal.

What not to do:

You don't want to set yourself up to feel guilty, and you don't want to let others down.

What to do:

1. Be certain that you are truly willing to do any task to which you commit yourself.

2. Be honest and strong with other people, especially friends and family, so that you say no if someone asks you to do something you don't want to do.

3. Assess yourself. How do you want to use your time on your day off? This may vary, so it will need to be done regularly.

4. If you want to "go with the flow," don't commit to doing a task at a specific time. Sometimes you may need to just hang out with people you like. Sometimes you may want to be alone. And sometimes you will feel like doing home repairs.

5. If you did tell someone you would do a chore and you later realize you don't want to do it, go to the person and explain how you feel. Don't just avoid that person. You're not asking permission not to do it. You're giving information.

6. If a chore is urgent, see if you can make it more bearable. For example, you may find that creating a "work crew" of friends who go from house to house makes chores tolerable as you combine camaraderie with the job.

7. If you have the resources, you may
    need to give yourself permission to
    hire someone to do the chore.

What makes this hard to do:

The cultural ethic that puts work before
play or relaxation may leave you feeling
guilty. You are neither *bad* nor irresponsible because you choose to do something you want to do. Simply express
your own value system and understand
that not everyone will like it. You need
not go along with what others believe is
right, but be kind and thoughtful as you
negotiate the practical matters of life.

View from the Cliff

LIMITING YOUR LOSSES

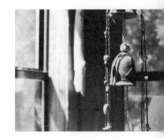

DO YOU REGULARLY BURN POTS, LOSE CONTACT LENSES, OR OVERFLOW THE BACKYARD POND BECAUSE YOU DON'T PAY ATTENTION TO WHAT YOU'RE DOING?

You turn on the stove, using a whistle-less teakettle to boil water. Or maybe you turn the water on full blast to fill the outside pond. Then you walk away to do something else while the task is being completed. After all, neither the teakettle nor pond needs your help to accomplish your goal. Staring at the water won't help heat it. But that's the last you think of it until you smell the dry kettle burning. You only notice you left the hose running after you see that the whole yard is flooded with water.

Maybe your challenge is finding a permanent solution to periodically dropping a contact lens while you're putting it in your eye. Rarely do you discover where it flew. And it costs you much money to ignore your inattentiveness.

All of the "pay attention to what you're doing" lectures do not work. But you want to stop endangering your home, wasting resources, and needlessly spending money.

Though you may not be able to solve your problem once and for all, you'd like to find a way to make the losses less frequent.

Why this happens:

- Any task that has a beginning and an end with nothing for you to do but wait in between means trouble. If you are an active person, doing nothing while you wait is next to impossible.

- If you do a task at intervals rather than repetitively, you will find it hard to develop a pattern that keeps attention focused during the waiting period.

- Cleaning a contact lens is a job that requires you to use only two fingers to rub the cleaning solution on the lens for a few seconds. Your eyes, ears, and other hand are free to do *something* during those seconds. It only takes a second or two, after all, to move things around in the medi-

cine cabinet. Or you start to wash the sink or put the cap back on the toothpaste. It's during the times of extra activity that you drop the lens or it flies out of your hand, never to be seen again.

What not to do:

Do not beat up on yourself or think you are irresponsible because your attention flags while you're waiting for something to finish getting done.

What to do:

1. Look for a solution that will reduce the frequency of your losses.

2. Believe it or not, there are actually people in the world who stand right by the stove while water comes to a boil or a pool fills. They even watch it. You are probably not one of them if The True You is a lively, creative person who enjoys doing many things.

3. Don't judge yourself. True, you need, for your own good, to learn to pay attention, but know it's as hard for slow-moving people to hurry as it is for active people to wait.

4. Decide upon one habit you'd like to change. Only work on one habit at a time. It will take a week or more to establish a habit to safeguard you against a particular loss.

5. You must discover something that will call your attention back onto the task during the period of waiting. This is quite individual. In the case of the boiling water, it could mean getting a kettle that whistles loudly. Then commit to immediately respond to the signal. If you ignore it, even for a short time, you will tune it out. Gentle timer beeps are far too easy to ignore and forget.

6. With a short task like contact lens cleaning, where you only have seconds to wait, you must commit to do *nothing* else. Though that is hard, try staring at your fingers and the lens that's being cleaned. Try counting to ten forwards or backwards. Smile to yourself, knowing you're instilling a money-saving habit. Do this for a week or two and you'll have habituated your behavior for a while at least. You'll probably need to reinforce this behavior every few months.

7. These kinds of solutions are likely to become habits *for a while*. They will require a refresher course periodically to reinforce something that is not natural. But that reminder won't take as long to reinstall, and you'll probably remember to pay attention for a longer period of time. You might want to schedule the repeater course by writing it on your calendar.

Following Through to Success

What makes this hard to do:

Establishing a habit that is not natural for you is difficult. Be patient with yourself. Solutions are not permanent, so remember to reinforce the habit regularly.

TUNING OUT

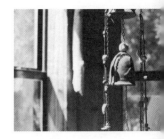

DO YOU SAY "UH-HUH" AND THEN FAIL TO FOLLOW THROUGH ON YOUR COMMITMENT?

Your coworker rolled her eyes at you today. She claims she told you that she needed a file that you have in your desk and you said, "Uh-huh." She expected you to bring it to her. You were in meetings all afternoon and didn't see her again until nearly five. When you returned, she said, "Where is the file you said you'd bring? I needed it this afternoon."

You said, "What file? You didn't ask for any file."

That's when she rolled her eyes. The worst part of is that it's not the first time something like this has happened. And your wife says you do the same thing at home—all the time.

You don't mean to do it. You're really not trying to avoid doing what they are asking of you. You even thought maybe you ought to have your hearing checked, but when you did, nothing was wrong. What's the deal?

Why this happens:

- Some people do a lot of thinking. Conversations run through their

79

heads and they watch movielike scenarios play out in their minds. If you're like this even a little bit, considerable time can go by with your attention focused inward.

■ If The True You is a big picture person who becomes wholly absorbed in what you're doing or thinking so that you become one with it, you may not perceive something said to you in a regular voice. This happens especially if you're busy or have a lot on your mind. It also happens if you have had a busy time and are now relaxing, watching TV, or meditating with your mind a million miles away.

■ Specifically, what happens is that you have a high enough level of attention to respond automatically with "Uh-huh," but not high enough to translate your response into action. You do not follow through because you didn't get the communication strongly enough to turn your agreement into action.

What not to do:

Do not continue to let other people down because of your level of attention.

What to do:

1. Be clear to those with whom you communicate about your attentional needs.

2. Enlist the assistance of each person with whom you have a relationship, business or personal. Tell the person that you may say "Uh-huh" to a request without registering the request strongly enough to do it. You may wish to add, "I'd very much like to do whatever you ask. I'd like to know when I tune out, but sometimes don't know I've done it, so I need your help."

3. Directly ask the person if he or she is willing to work with you. By asking for help, you are being responsible for your difficulty. If someone, usually an angry spouse, says he's tired

of your dependency and refuses to work with you, know that there is more wrong with the relationship than this one issue. Also realize the individual is struggling with his or her problems and issues. Don't accept his scolding or criticism, and don't expect the person to be able to be on your team.

4. Suggest a willing helper (secretary, spouse, or friend) stop you when he or she needs something from you. It doesn't matter if it's a file or taking out the garbage. Tell the person to touch you, call your name, or have you repeat the request. Suggest the person ask, "What did I just tell you?" or "When will you bring me the file?" or "When will you take out the trash?" Each of these questions calls for more direct attention from you and will nudge you to a deeper level of attention. You can expect that the questions be asked nicely, not with an exasperated tone.

Interestingly, if you're asked right away, "What did I say?" you'll be able to answer even though your focus was elsewhere. But if even a second or two pass, you won't be able to recall the request. With the early query, you'll be able to break into your thinking or reverie and your awareness of the request will be heightened. Then you'll remember to do it.

5. The examples talked about here assume you're willing to respond to the request and are not using "Uh-huh" as a diversionary tactic to get someone off your back. It's up to you to follow through on the request immediately.

6. Say, "Thank you, I appreciate your helping me with this." The problem may not get better over time but it need not cause trouble with a team approach.

What makes this hard to do:

If you or someone else feels you are being irresponsible and blames or shames you for your lack of awareness, you are likely to get into arguments. Bad feelings and emotional sparring will likely take the place of genuine teamwork. Don't engage in this nonconstructive behavior.

ANCHORING A DRIFTING MIND

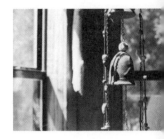

DOES YOUR MIND EVER DRIFT FROM WHAT YOU ARE READING OR FROM SOMEONE WHO IS SPEAKING TO YOU?

You are reading and the next thing you know you're at the bottom of the page and don't have a clue what you just read. Your mind also drifts when you are listening to someone speak to you. It happens when the person speaks to you directly or when you are in an audience or group. You've noticed you have particular trouble if the other person doesn't get to the point quickly enough to hold your attention.

Why this happens:

■ As a person whose brain focuses on the interconnections and relationships between things more than on specific bits of information, you are likely to drift away from one thought to a complex of thoughts. That's just how you are made. You quickly and automatically connect what you hear with what you already know.

■ Something we read, see, hear, or otherwise perceive draws our attention to think about or feel about it as it applies to us. This happens when you are a kinesthenic learner. You become very involved in what you are doing and *begin to live* the experience. So if you are reading about geology, you may begin to think about how much you like turquoise and how you'd like to go to Arizona to learn to do silversmithing so you can make jewelry.

- You may also begin to have feelings that pull you off track. For example, your boss is telling you about your next assignment, and you begin to feel scared that you won't be able to accomplish it. You become all tied up in your feelings of fear and your mind stops listening to what your boss is saying.

- You may become bored, already knowing what the writer or speaker is going to say. Taking too long to get to the point annoys you. Worse yet, your mind drifts as you think about other things, waiting for the sentence to end.

- You become distracted by your own body's needs or by something you see or hear in the environment.

What not to do:

Please don't beat up on yourself or feel helpless because your mind drifts.

What to do:

1. Learn to anchor your attention so you won't stay "off track" for a long time.

2. Begin to tell yourself that you can develop the skill of noticing when your mind drifts.

3. If you are reading and your mind drifts, place your finger on the place in the book where you begin to think about something other than what you are reading. This will take a little practice to catch yourself in a timely manner.

4. In the column of your book or on a nearby notepaper you keep handy for such purposes, jot a word or two down or draw a picture that will remind you of your intervening thought. You may want to note the place in the reading where the thought occurs.

5. Commit to return to your note later.

6. Promise to honor your creative thinking by paying attention to your notes after you finish reading. Be sure to follow through on this commitment.

7. If your mind drifts during a conversation, ask the person to repeat what was just said. There is nothing wrong with this. If you ask with confidence, it's usually perceived as a compliment. You can even mention your mind drifted. Say, "I started thinking about what you were talking about and need you to repeat the next thing you said. I don't want to miss anything you said."

8. Begin repeating what the person is saying to yourself.

9. If you begin to feel an emotion that is distracting you, note the feeling instantly and return your attention to what is being said to you. Promise yourself you'll deal with your feelings later.

10. Nod your head slightly to the speaker, affirming to yourself that you are paying attention. Look the speaker in the eye. Occasionally repeat what the speaker just said for clarification.

11. As a member of an audience, ask for clarification as soon as you fail to understand because you began to think of something else. Say, "Excuse me for interrupting. I want to be sure I understand what you are saying." Realize you're giving the speaker a compliment.

12. If you're becoming bored, grit your teeth, play a rhythmic tune with

your toes on the inside of your shoe, or do anything else that's quiet to help you pass the time. Remind yourself to "pay attention." If you know the person well, you can say, "I truly understand what you're saying. I'm eager to hear your next thought."

13. If your body's needs are distracting you because you're hungry or tired of sitting or you are noticing some other discomfort, pat yourself and say reassuringly to yourself that you'll take care of the need as soon as possible. If you know the person reasonably well, you might interject, "I want to hear what you're saying, but my stomach is growling. Can we get a snack while we're talking?"

14. If you're distracted by an outside interference, you may wish to request a change that will reduce the distraction, such as closing the door. Also focus on the speaker's mouth as if you're reading lips and tell your-

self, "I only have to focus for a little longer. I can do it."

15. When you're listening to a speaker rather than engaged in dialogue, have something in your hands that can stimulate your alertness, such as a paper clip, handiwork, or a pencil and paper on which to doodle or take notes.

16. Make your own personal variations on these tips. But know that, with a little practice on your part, you can learn to anchor your attention at a much higher level than you now do.

What makes this hard to do:

It takes practice to get through to your attention to learn new habits. You must tell yourself you can do it. *And you must practice for a while.*

Whenever possible, avoid truly boring situations.

View from the Cliff

RETURNING TO COLLEGE

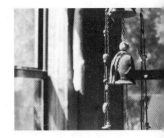

ARE YOU WORRIED THAT YOU'LL NEVER BE ABLE TO GET THE HIGHER EDUCATION YOU NEED TO DO WHAT YOU WANT TO DO IN LIFE?

Right out of high school you tried college but dropped out after one semester with terrible grades. Now several years later, you want to help people, but to be allowed to do that, you must return to school. You're terrified the same thing will happen. Without a college degree, however, you won't be able to go farther on the career path you've found—one you enjoy and want to follow for a long time.

Book work has always been really difficult for you. You learn by doing, not by reading books, writing papers, and taking tests. You wish there was an apprenticeship that would teach you everything you need to know.

Why this happens:

■ As a sensitive, big picture, kines-thenic-learning person who takes in everything at once, entering any new educational level can be overwhelming. That's part of what happened to you after high school. You went from a fairly structured environment where you were told what, when, and how to do most things to an unstructured, chaotic, demanding one that required you to build your own structure out of a mass of options.

You not only had to take into account your course work, but all the requirements for living. That's two major jobs. Add to that the fact that you probably changed your social group and your support network. That's enough to overwhelm anyone with a brainstyle like yours.

- When you first went to college without a clear picture of where you were headed, you faced way too many options to sort through them all in the short time you had to get organized. Confusion was a likely result.

- College programs teach students using only a fraction of the forms of intelligence available for learning. They favor linear learners who can memorize facts and take tests well. If you're not a person who handles details easily and you learn by working in a kinesthenic (apprenticeship) way, practicing what you're learning, you are likely to have trouble with higher education. At least, you won't work up to your level of intellectual potential.

- The first time a kinesthenic, sensitive, big picture person tackles a large new enterprise, the results often are less than wonderful. But after you've run through the routine—remember, being kinesthenic, you learn by doing—you will have a much clearer idea of what to expect and how to handle the situation. You will be familiar with how to accomplish many of the tasks that face you. As a result, you'll actually have much less work to do the second time around.

What not to do:

Do not panic that you'll have a repeat performance of an earlier failure.

What to do:

1. Follow your dreams to continue your education.

2. Note the difference in yourself since you first attempted college.

3. Start a journal or a conversation with another person about your college voyage. A mentor or someone who believes in you can be an enormous asset at this time. Continue to write or talk about your current goals and reasons for going to college now.

4. Look for colleges and training programs that are nontraditional, inventive, and offer "credit for experience" programs. You may find guides in the resource section of your public library and in high school counseling offices. Community colleges often serve as excellent institutions to begin higher education.

5. Talk with a new student counselor or a counselor for students with special needs. Returning students fall into this category.

6. Utilize the Americans with Disabilities Act. You are likely to qualify if you're a big picture, kinesthenic learner who is more intelligent than your school performance has shown. Realize that what you need is an equal opportunity to learn what you're capable of learning and prove what you know. (See the addendum at the end of this chapter for details.)

7. Whether you use the Americans with Disabilities Act or not, take small classes and a light class load, especially at first.

8. Don't worry about grades. Instead, keep focused on getting the degree, the power credential, and on getting out of school so you can do what you want to do.

9. Stay focused on one semester or quarter at a time. Though you will occasionally need or want to look at the big picture, that can get overwhelming, so don't do it very often. Take college one step at a time.

10. Select your professors carefully—be sure to choose those who teach using communication methods that you understand. If you get into a class in which you can't understand what's going on, withdraw immediately and search for a different professor you *can* understand. The presentation style of a teacher can make the difference between failing or passing a class.

11. Get to know the professors and teachers in your areas of interest.

Often they can help you from behind the scenes to get through classes that are difficult for you.

12. Seriously consider using tutors and study groups.

13. Consider finding ways to work in the job area that interests you while you are in school. This will reinforce your interests and will help you stay motivated in the tough classes. You also are likely to find mentors in job settings who will encourage you.

14. Be sure to have some fun and R & R along the way. Even consider taking a break for a semester unless you feel you won't go back. You know yourself. Follow your sense about this suggestion.

What makes this hard to do:

Because much college work for a kinesthenic learner is like trying to run a marathon with a fifty-pound weight on each leg, you may become discouraged. If you do, take a little time off. Also consider other avenues that will allow you to do what you love. There is often more than one route to your goal. You may need to change majors rather than giving up your dream.

The Americans with Disabilities Act

- You must realize that what you need to get through school is an equal opportunity to learn what you're capable of learning and to prove you know it.

- Currently that means you will need to turn to the Americans with Disabilities Act (ADA). This act says that if you have the intelligence to learn a subject but have some learning difficulties that get in the way of applying that intelligence, you must be given reasonable accommodation so you can succeed.

- You need to go to the Special Services Office at the college to initiate the process and determine your eligibility. You can do this even before classes start.

- To formally acquire ADA accommodation, you must undergo an assessment of your intellectual capability. You must also be assessed with regard to your "handicapping condition." If there is sufficient discrepancy between these two assessments, you are "diagnosed" with what is called a learning disability. Many of the difficulties kinesthenic, big picture people have in school lead to the assignment of a learning disabilities label such as ADD or ADHD. With this label you can apply for special services at your school of choice.

  The testing must be done by a licensed professional such as a psychologist or psychiatrist. Sometimes an educational diagnostician's or counselor's testing is acceptable.

- Many college offices are now working with professors and students in an attempt to provide learner-friendly approaches and materials for all students without the need of formal testing.

- Some of the services available include:

Unlimited test-taking time

A quiet area, free of distraction, in which to take tests

Tests designed to support the brain-style construction of students, i.e., essays, projects, oral exams, instead of multiple choice or fill-in-the-blank formats

Assignment of a note taker

Assistance in outlining main points in class and textbook material

Use of a tape recorder during lectures

One-on-one tutoring

Front-row seating

Priority use of computer resources designed to help students with organization and study skills

Access to recorded versions of text-books

Assistance in creating a structured time schedule

Assistance in developing priorities for long-term projects

Assistance in relating to authority figures

Assistance in translating differences in brainstyles

Substitution of a required class with one that isn't compromised because of the learning difference

These are only some of the services available—a student may request any reasonable accommodation.

■ You need to know that you can request these accommodations whether you're formally identified as learning disabled or as someone with an ADD style of brain construction not favored in school. More and more college teachers, especially at the community college level, are responding to students' learning needs.

■ However, without a formal diagnosis, the faculty is not *mandated* to provide what you need.

What makes this hard to do:

You must be honest with yourself and not attempt to use ADA so that you can study subject matter that is not suited to your overall capability.

ADA requires you to say that you are "disabled" when in reality that is a misnomer. What you need is simply the opportunity to do your work in a way that fits you. Ultimately, this right will be seen as the diversity issue that it is and, as a result, will fall under equal opportunities legislation. Then you will not have to say you're handicapped in order to be given the opportunity to get an education or do your job. But for now, ADA can make a difference in your life.

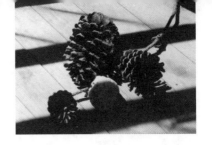

PART THREE

Behaving Yourself

If I am not for myself, who is for me?
And when I am for myself, what am
I? And if not now, when?

HILLEL

30 B.C.–A.D. 10

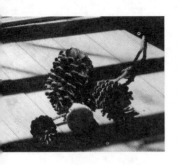

Often the style of our brain construction dictates the kinds of behaviors we struggle to overcome. In this chapter you'll learn that there is not one right way to be or do things in order to get what you want. You'll find ways that can work for you because they follow the nature of The True You.

Temper, impulsivity, and getting a "high" are all behaviors that make foreheads crease with a scowl. These and many other behaviors fall outside the limits of acceptable social conduct. Yet these are forms of communication that carry a message of need. For example, instead of using words to express "I'm afraid. I need to feel protected," a temper outburst surrounds a person with a layer of protection, creating an illusion of safety.

But the price of unacceptable behavior is high, and the efficiency of meeting the actual inner need is low. When The True You is naturally active, verbally, mentally, and physically, you are also likely to find that your behavior spills over the boundaries of acceptable behavior.

What a relief to become aware of some of the many opportunities to gain not only clarity into why you behave as you do, but options to get your needs met without incurring a high price tag. Learning to stay true to yourself while remaining within the parameters established by social limits allows you to win along all fronts in the best interest of yourself and those around you.

You'll learn to live in a world that

requires self-responsibility, communication, and thoughtfulness of others even when it also demands that you accommodate it in ways that don't readily fit you. Living according to the values in which you believe will stop further personal wounding as well as wounding of others as you take charge of your behavior. The Accommodating You can and will discover how to bridge the difference.

The True You, working with The Accommodating You, will find ways to hold down your end of a task while finding ways to support your style of brain construction. You'll be able to let others know what you need and what you can give. Everyone ends up a winner.

HANDLING CHANGE

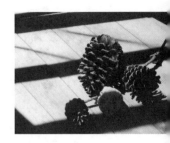

DO YOU DISLIKE CHANGE, MOSTLY BECAUSE YOU FALL APART WHEN YOU ARE CONFRONTED WITH IT?

You recently took a new job and you wonder whether you'll ever catch on, much less get caught up with all you have to do. Meanwhile you're trying to bring order into a new house. You are trying to help your kids get settled in school. And you want to do something about filling in the void created by leaving old friends.

Seems like every time your life changes, you feel awful and fall apart.

You need extra sleep, become tearful over the littlest things, and even have more health problems than usual. You get short with your family, are sure you've made a horrible mistake, and feel that you will probably get fired and be out on the street in days.

Why this happens:

- As a big picture, kinesthenic person who takes in everything around you *all at once,* you suffer enormous overload when you are confronted with changes. Everything is new.

- When The True You lives by patterns—that is, the relationships between things more than details—change brings problems. It creates a breakup of the old patterns that guided you. In addition, it takes you a while to see the new patterns because they are made of a lot of details. To establish new habits and integrate them into new patterns takes time. So you are left initially with no way to structure what you are experiencing.

- As someone who doesn't organize according to details, often not knowing what to initially do with individual occurrences, you are suddenly attacked by a myriad of new things.

- If you're sensitive, you will *feel* your discomfort intensely.

- To the degree to which you take things personally, you may think that what is happening to you is personal. You may feel as if you are the only one who gets so upset, reacts so poorly, or feels so badly.

- All change causes all people to have to adjust.

- When change happens *to* you, it's usually more unsettling than if you create it.

- Change is cumulative. If you've had a lot of change recently, you are likely to have failed to recover from early stresses before incurring new ones. Pretty soon you're awash in stress.

What not to do:

Do not rush into your new situation and ignore your need to let your body, mind, and emotions adjust at their own rate.

What to do:

1. Learn to handle the results of change so you learn from them rather than get wounded by them.

2. At first, simplify your life by only doing exactly what you *have* to do.

3. Get extra hours of sleep. Be sure to eat healthy food regularly. Take refreshing breaks (naps) even when it means you don't get things done.

4. Do not rush. Do not take on new tasks or try to be creative until you've stabilized your life.

5. Spend time considering what you have to do and what you want to do. Making a list helps a lot of us to get all the new details out of our heads. But don't think you have to accomplish the whole list at once. Be cautious not to become overwhelmed because, as a big picture person, you see everything you have to do.

6. Take some time to set priorities. Maybe time with your family comes first. Learning your new job comes next. Time for yourself may follow. Next work on your new home.

Hanging pictures may be way down the list, as are other nonessentials, unless you feel adrift without them.

7. Most people rush, thinking they must get everything organized in the first month or so. It takes a minimum of six months to a year to rebalance big life changes. If you've also undergone a loss (such as a divorce or death), it will take closer to two to three years.

8. If, for whatever reason, your change does not turn out to be satisfactory after you've given yourself time to adjust, don't stay stuck just because of concern for what others might think. Even if you initiated the change, move on. There's little way of knowing how things will work out until you live with the choices you make. Resist the adage, "You made your bed, now lie in it." Remember, kinesthenic learners learn by doing, that is, trying out situations. Only then can we tell how something will

work for us and how we will feel about it.

What makes this hard to do:

Most people rush through change, failing to realize how strenuous it is.

Family and friends may insert their opinions regarding your adjustment period. Tell them, "Thank you," then do what your mind, body, and emotions are telling you is the right thing to do for you at a given time.

TAKING CONTROL OF YOUR IMPULSIVITY

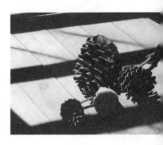

DO YOU DO THINGS WITHOUT THINKING?

On a hot summer day you're working in the kitchen with your mother. She sighs and you notice her perspiring. Impulsively, you reach to get a water glass out of the cupboard. You don't take the time to watch what you're doing and you knock it over, causing it to fall and break on the counter. Your mother clucks her tongue at your clumsiness.

This kind of thing happens to you a lot. Only a few days ago you were hurrying downstairs when you noticed a pile of clothes on the landing awaiting transport to the basement for washing. Impulsively, you changed direction so you could pick up the clothes. You caught your rubber sole on the stair edge and fell. Fortunately, you caught yourself on the railing or you might have taken a nasty spill. You'd sure like a quarter for every impulsive move you've made in your life.

Why this happens:

- Driven by feelings more than thoughts, you may try to please someone or take care of something by quickly doing whatever you feel will help.

- If you have a long-standing habit of short-changing yourself by focusing on others exclusively, forgetting what you need, you will likely act impulsively and suffer as a result. Suffering wounds you.

- Your sensitivity to another's needs may drive you to do something before you've had time to think through a plan of action and implement it.

- To the degree to which The True You is a kinesthenic person, a doer, you'll tend to find your solutions by acting them out. You really don't learn by being told what to do. Instead, you learn from experience, unless you're shamed, which increases anxiety and sets you up to act even more impulsively. Left unassaulted by shame, you probably won't fail to look when reaching in a cupboard the next time.

- Impulsivity tends to be present when you feel you cannot get what you need. As a result, when you see even a tiny opening on the pathway to get what you need, you jump at it.

- It's not so much that you're innately clumsy. It's more that you're quickly trying to do two or more things at once. For example, you're reacting to your feelings *and* taking action at the same time.

What not to do:

Do not continue to let your impulsive tendencies express themselves unchecked.

What to do:

1. Know you can get your needs met while honoring The True You. If The Wounded You feels fearful in this respect, say to yourself, "I'll learn to get my needs met without hurting myself."

View from the Cliff

2. Envision yourself as someone who has a natural rhythm—one that can smoothly and skillfully guide you through your daily activities.

3. Recall how you were raised, and refashion your beliefs about yourself if necessary to achieve a new, positive self-image. See yourself as coordinated rather than clumsy, or spontaneously helpful rather than impulsive.

4. Affirm to yourself that you can learn to get your actions under your control. You may wish to say, "I can get my actions under control," or "I can control my actions."

5. Practice taking a breath before you act.

6. Look for specific triggers that cue you to act. One common trigger is trying to please someone else. Another trigger is feeling ashamed or inadequate. By analyzing past impulsive acts, you will begin to be more aware of the emotional or situational triggers that get you in trouble. As you become more aware, you can head off action and keep it under your control.

7. To deal with a trigger such as wanting to please another person, tell yourself that it's okay to want to please someone else, but not at your expense.

8. Congratulate yourself for even the smallest improvement. Taking one step at a time will get you where you want to go.

What makes this hard to do:

Lack of awareness of the emotional and situational triggers that precede impulsive acts makes it hard to change impulsive behavior. Habits, long ago formed, take time to change.

SHIFTING GEARS AND BEING INTERRUPTED

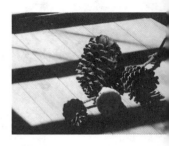

DOES IT DRIVE YOU CRAZY TO HAVE TO CHANGE FROM ONE TASK TO ANOTHER OR BE INTERRUPTED WHEN YOU ARE INVOLVED IN A TASK?

Whether you're working on a computer, organizing your kitchen, or doing any of a thousand other jobs, you may dislike being interrupted. Maybe you even blow up. After all, you've learned it's hard, if not impossible, to begin again where you left off. You also have trouble shifting from one task to another on your own. Once you've started something, you hate to stop until you are done. You may even pull all-nighters, oblivious to your physical needs for food and sleep, ignoring calls to dinner or bed.

Why this happens:

- The attention regulator in your brain tends to have two settings, on and off. There's no in between. So it's difficult to readily shift from one thing to another when you're interrupted or the task requires you to change direction.

- You also are likely to see the big picture, the completed project you're working on. You may see the "best possible scenario" for whatever you are doing. You want to get to these projections before you quit working.

- You may be able to do only one thing at a time. It could even be hard for you to deal with more than one relationship at a time.

What not to do:

Don't blow up or blow a task off because you have trouble shifting gears when you are interrupted or need to change direction.

What to do:

1. Engage in self-study. Be aware of your reactions to being interrupted or changing tasks. Do you feel stressed under these conditions? Has it always been hard for you, even in childhood? Have you tended to do one thing at a time? Have you tended to have one relationship at a time? Do you do better concentrating on only one subject or task until it is completed, rather than juggling several at a time?

2. Because transition times are often very difficult for you, you need to be particularly aware of any demands coming from outside of your current focus.

3. When your needs are different from others', explain how you work and then set specific limits on yourself, allowing extra time to change from one task to another.

   For example, if you are organizing your kitchen during the day but plan to go out to dinner in the evening, you'll need to allow extra time to stop your daytime activity. You'll need extra time for the transition required to clean up and change clothes. It's up to you to take responsibility to stop *on time* rather than expecting another person to have to wait for you.

4. Once you've committed to a reasonable schedule, make plans for how to mark the place where you stopped. This could, for example, be a red bow on the kitchen cabinet you just worked on. It might be a list with completed items crossed off using a colored pen. Or you might lay the pen across the line on the list where you want to return to work.

5. Reassure yourself that you'll complete your task by setting the time when you'll return to it.

6. Explain to anyone you're involved with about your need to stay with a task. Tell the person how you'll help them to remember. Say, "I'll put up a sign that says, 'No interrupting, please.'" Or say, gently, "Not now. I'll be taking a break at two o'clock." Or, "Can we talk tomorrow?" Ask others not to disturb your uncom-

pleted project. Thank them in advance and again later for helping you, so they understand how important it is to you.

7. If you are in a situation such as a timed exam that requires you to quickly shift from one section to another, you may need to ask for accommodation to take the sections separately, allowing time for transition from one to another. (See the section about the Americans with Disabilities Act, p. 91.)

What makes this hard to do:

You are likely to suffer greatly if you try to follow anyone else's time frame. You may even find it impossible because it's so hard for you to get back on task after being interrupted. As a result you may have developed habits, such as blowing up, that take time to revise. But you can do it.

HAVING A TEMPER OUTBURST

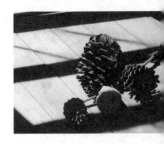

ARE YOU KNOWN FOR HAVING A TEMPER?

The special person in your life is having a birthday. Though you hate shopping, you want very much to find just the right present. You even turned down an opportunity to spend time with friends to take the time to shop. You find the store jammed with people, and there are no clerks to be found to help you. finally you find something you think your friend will like but not in the size you need. You make your way to the service counter so you can ask if they have others in the back. The person says he has no time to check. Something inside of you snaps, and you tell the clerk off. Then you stomp out of the store empty-handed.

Why this happens:

- Anyone can have a temper outburst when under enough stress. A temper display is protective covering for feelings of helplessness and vulnerability. It may happen when you don't get something you badly want or are hurt or startled.

- People who are sensitive are vulnerable and more likely to get hurt, so they often throw up a temper shield for protection.

- Temper expressions can become habits. When your temper outburst has provided you with what you wanted, having a temper outburst easily becomes a habit. Even when you've been repeatedly scolded for blowing up, your temper was reinforced and became habituated. The problem is that the price of having a temper is high, even when you get a payoff, because tempers are exhausting. Also, other people may get tired of being around your temper displays and scold you. They may even begin to reject you.

- Kinesthenic people act out their anger tangibly in observable ways, such as slamming doors, yelling, cursing, and driving too fast. If you are a kinesthenic person, you run a high likelihood of having an observable temper.

- If you fear you will not get your basic needs met, you may cover your fear with a temper outburst.

What not to do:

Do not continue to allow yourself to let your temper control you.

What to do:

1. Make a pledge to yourself that you'll find new ways to self-protect and get your needs met.

2. Think about the last time your temper got out of control.

3. Ask yourself what happened immediately before your outburst. That event served as a trigger for your temper. You will be able to use this awareness to head off further temper outbursts.

4. Everyone has specific "hot buttons." When these are touched, even lightly, you are more vulnerable to react

strongly. If you have an especially strong need to please others, you'll be more susceptible to situations that get in the way of your gaining that approval.

Or if you are fearful that someone won't accept you unless you please them by getting the right thing for them, you are in a position to lose a lot of emotional security. This is a setup for a temper outburst.

5. To curb your temper, make a purposeful decision to work on it. This means finding ways to attend to the inner needs that lie behind your temper.

6. Become watchful of situations that trigger your temper. Especially notice when you're feeling stressed, are in a hurry, or are fearful of an outcome. Maybe you're hungry or lonely or tired.

7. Bring your hidden needs out in the open. Tell someone you can confide in about them. You may need to do some counseling work at this point. Know it takes courage to face your inner vulnerabilities. But the reward is worth it.

8. You may also make a list of other ways to protect yourself besides blowing up.

9. If someone feeds your temper by giving in to you or nagging and scolding you when you blow up, tell that person you are working to change and ask them to refrain. They may or may not be able to respect your request.

10. Only you can be responsible for stopping your temper behavior. But if you're being reinforced by someone, you may have to decide to back away from that person if they can't stop reinforcing your nonconstructive habit.

11. Congratulate yourself when you

make headway. Though expecting perfection right away is not realistic, watch for little gains and be proud of yourself.

What makes this hard to do:

The hardest part of getting a temper under control is dealing with someone who sabotages your progress by being involved with your temper demands. You may also find tough going if you believe you can't get your needs met except by having a temper outburst.

DISPLACING YOUR TEMPER ONTO OTHERS

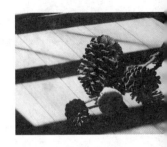

DO YOU DISPLACE YOUR ANGER ON PEOPLE YOU LOVE?

You work for a boss who treats her employees unfairly. You'd like to tell her off, but you're afraid you'll lose your job, so you swallow your feelings. But this approach is causing you to lose your temper in other settings. For example, when you're driving, you yell at other drivers. Worse yet, you're starting to become irritable with the people you love, and for the littlest things. You know you need to get your temper under control.

Why this happens:

■ If you are in a situation where you can get in trouble because you are angry at a person, especially an authority, you, like most of us, are likely to bottle up your temper. Parents, bosses, teachers, and police are examples of such authorities.

■ But the anger doesn't go away because you've kept it inside. If anything, it actually becomes stronger.

■ When you are with someone you do

not fear or with whom you have no connection, the bottled-up anger is likely to come out. Kicking the dog, fighting with someone weaker than you, or snapping at a stranger such as a clerk are examples of this. Road rage reflects displacement of anger. You see it when someone shoots the finger at you for a driving infraction or cuts in and out of traffic, coming dangerously close to accidents with other drivers. These are extremely dangerous situations, and the best advice is to get as far away from the angry person as you can.

What not to do:

Do not displace your anger on others, spreading your temper.

What to do:

1. Do get back in charge of your life and your emotions.

2. Recognize what you're doing and commit to stop displacing your

anger onto other people and situations.

3. Pay attention to the cause of your anger. That's what you have to work on.

4. Assess whether you can work out the situation that is causing you to become angry. Ask yourself if you think you can rectify the situation if you talk in a professional or calm manner. Knowing about the problem, the individual may be able to change. Other times, the person may not be able to change. But it's worth a try. Approach the person calmly with a plan for how to change the situation. Always have a plan to suggest, rather than just going to the person to complain.

5. When you're in a situation that is destructive, you can expect to feel angry. Assess the cost of staying in it if no changes are possible. Caution

must be used whether you decide to stay or leave it.

6. Rationally consider what would happen if you leave the situation. Notice whether your reactions are based on fear. Notice if you feel relieved when you think about leaving. No situation is worth your emotional health and well-being. There are always other opportunities available to you.

7. If you're afraid to make a change, evaluate how you see yourself. Ask yourself whether you are afraid of failure. Do you see yourself as inadequate? If so, work on this. Your feelings belie the truth of your potential and the wonder of what you have to offer, but you may have to learn this.

8. Until you either resolve the issue or are able to leave the hurtful situation, consider ways to turn your angry energy into something constructive, either at work or outside, instead of displacing it where it doesn't belong. For example, you may become competitive, generating additional business on the job. You might channel your emotions into inventive and creative challenges as you focus on problems that have gone unsolved. You may express your anger artistically. Consider physically working off your energy by running, engaging in athletics, chopping wood, digging in the garden, or pursuing strenuous activity. But remember, this is only temporary until you get yourself out of the destructive situation.

What makes this hard to do:

To get back in charge of your life, you'll need to resolve old emotional issues that caused you pain in the past and will cause you to face that pain now. You'll also have to change long-standing habits. These are hard jobs, but not unbearable ones, and the results are well worth the effort on your part.

LIVING WITH UNEXPRESSED TEMPER

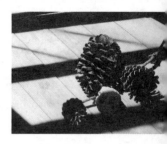

DO YOU FEEL AT A LOSS ABOUT WHAT TO DO WHEN YOU CAN'T SAFELY EXPRESS YOUR ANGRY FEELINGS?

You are confined or trapped in a situation without the option of leaving—one over which you feel you have no tangible power or choice. You've always had a bad temper, but if you lose it now, you'll either be punished or will feel terribly guilty. You live with a high level of fear, never knowing when your temper will go off.

Why this happens:

■ Being confined in a situation means you have no tangible power, no matter how powerful you were at earlier times or how emotionally powerful you may still be. This leads to a high level of stress.

■ Being trapped in a situation that you simply can't give yourself permission to leave, such as caring for a chronically ill family member, places enormous pressure on you. It creates feelings of helplessness.

- Feeling helpless or vulnerable is one of the underlying reasons for a temper to be triggered. Your fear of a temper outburst is well taken if you will either get in trouble or feel terrible if you discharge the temper. In this situation, you are faced with the need to find alternative ways to survive.

What not to do:

Do not think your situation is hopeless.

What to do:

1. Because you do not have the option of leaving your situation and have limited ways to channel your energy, you must quickly learn to do something with your temper.

2. You have a golden opportunity to face the underlying causes for your reactions. So your first step is to look deeply within yourself to the source of your fear, helplessness, hopelessness, and frustration—feelings that feed your temper.

3. Be gentle but tenacious with your explorations.

4. You may want to try writing your feelings down. Or you may find talking them out with another person or in a group is more to your liking. You may decide to seek counseling to explore the feelings and memories that underlie your temper.

5. Often temper tantrums start in childhood, raging unrestrained from then on. Recall, as best you can, a time when, as a child, you had a temper tantrum.

6. As you visualize that child part of you in your mind or recall the scene, ask what you needed at the time. Do not chide yourself for wanting or needing something then, even if all your memories are of people telling you that you shouldn't need it.

7. Begin to think about alternative ways to help that child part of you get what you wanted and needed.

8. Rewrite the early scenario in your mind or in a journal, seeing your grown-up self helping your child part get what was needed without throwing a temper tantrum.

9. Continue to raise that child part of yourself, showing options so that your child part has more than one way to get your needs met, even currently in a difficult situation. Be very self-nurturing. Commit to staying with the child part of you.

10. Project your new imagery technique for getting your needs met into some future scenario so that you'll have some practice in constructively facing future situations when they occur. Mentally practice conquering the kinds of situations that used to get you in trouble. Even as you're confronted with a currently stressful situation that taxes you, acknowledge inwardly to the child part of you that you understand the stress and will stay with your child part. Say you are sending support.

You will notice that you experience a lightening of the pressure within you. It doesn't fix or even change the external situation, but it does change the effect on you, giving you relief and perspective.

What makes this hard to do:

The hardest part of changing the habit of a hot temper is not believing you'll be able to learn constructive ways to get what you want and need. Because you learned helplessness in this regard from a very young age, it will take time and practice to learn new habits. But you can do it!

RESPONDING TO DISRESPECT

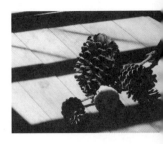

DOES IT MAKE YOU SO ANGRY WHEN SOMEONE TREATS YOU OR A LOVED ONE WITH DISRESPECT THAT YOU GO ON THE OFFENSIVE?

Recently, when you were on vacation, you and your companion spent the afternoon seeing the sights. You were enjoying yourself until a guard yelled sharply, "Time to go." You weren't quite through looking at one exhibit. It would only take a couple of minutes to finish, so you kept looking, knowing you'd leave soon. But the guard came right up next to you and said loudly, "I told you, we're closing! Get going!"

Not only did he get in your companion's face, but he reached toward you to guide you to the exit. You feared he was going to use force, and you'd have to resist him.

You felt extremely angry and yelled at him. Your friend became afraid you'd end up in trouble if you didn't keep your mouth shut. But your strong feelings that people ought to act respectfully toward others made it really hard to remain still. If he needed you to leave so quickly, he could have said so in a regular voice, perhaps even saying he understood that it's frustrating to be interrupted when you're viewing something of interest. Though you wouldn't have wanted to leave, you wouldn't have gotten angry.

You have the same reaction when someone scolds or criticizes you or anyone else for that matter. You hate it!

Why this happens:

■ As a sensitive person who feels everything keenly, you will tend to feel deeply about anything in which you place value. This includes the belief that people ought to treat each other with respect.

■ Being ordered to do something instead of being asked is overkill when you are a person who is loyal, sensitive, and has a good track record. It feels insulting and tends to create a need to throw up a defensive shield to cover hurt. When you're simply asked to do something, it's amazing how cooperative you and people like you become.

■ If you tend to be a feelings person, you lead with your feelings, feeling first, thinking later. Even though some of your buddies may be able to brush this kind of thing off, you will take it personally and *feel* terrible about it. (See Taking Things Personally, p. 178.)

■ To the degree to which you are a people-pleaser, you will try to do the best you can for anyone you admire. But if you don't admire another's behavior, you either get depressed or want to retaliate.

■ If you are self-monitoring, then you feel awful when someone judges or evaluates you or another person, and you want to fight back.

What not to do:

Do not overreact or openly respond to a troublesome situation until you have had time to think how you want to handle it.

What to do:

1. Learn to look at situations with some perspective, as if you are watching what is happening from a distance.

2. Clearly distinguish between your personal feelings and the event. This requires you to use your thinking mind in conjunction with your feelings.

3. To do this, become aware of what you're feeling. Do nothing about it at first. Just get clear.

4. Now engage your thinking mind and review what happened to kick off your feelings.

5. Analyze what might be happening to the other person. Maybe he is zealous about his job, fearful he will not do it well enough. Maybe she's always been treated harshly and doesn't know any other way to treat people. Maybe she was never treated with respect. Maybe his job power has gone to his head.

6. Find ways to self-protect that won't get you in trouble, such as whispering your irritation to your companion. Or you might compose a letter to the person's boss, telling about the incident. Include suggestions of a better way to handle the situation. You might also make jokes about the situation after you leave. The stand-up comic in you may have found great resource material.

7. Know what kind of power you have. No matter how wonderful your value system or how honest, forthright, or cooperative you are, others can't tell that until they get to know you. If they have more tangible power than you, you'll need to concede to them, at least until they can get to know you. Anyone, even an emotionally powerless person who has more job-related power than you, will have power *over* you. You need to factor

this in when you're deciding what to do.

8. If you're dealing with someone who has authority over you or someone who is not interpersonally insightful, you may want to choose to say nothing. But assess what the person can handle and then decide if you want to work with the issue.

9. To defend yourself against the pain of being ordered about, criticized, or scolded, check to see whether you asked for the input or not. Be cautious not to ask someone for help or ask for an opinion unless you're willing to take whatever they give you. A lot of people think that a request means you *want* criticism. Let the person know clearly what you want from them.

   By the way, it's okay to ask for someone to tell you your work is wonderful. Say, "I don't want criticism. Just tell me what this piece says to you."

If someone is demanding, scolding, or critical, you can simply say, "I don't appreciate what you're saying." Then back off. Unwanted criticism is something you have control over.

10. If a person with whom you are in contact regularly continues to use a scolding tone with you, know that some people sound that way because of their past experience. They may not even know they sound that way. You can feel sorry for the person, which will help you feel better. You can ask, "Are you intending to scold me?" If the person says no, continue, "I feel as if you are." Consider adding, "I don't do well when I'm scolded or criticized. I'd appreciate your not doing it."

   Own up to any errors, saying, "Though I may have made a mistake or didn't do something the way you would have liked me to do it, I'm not willing to be scolded for it. You can tell me what you want. I'll do my best." Your own tone needs to be moderate and free of scolding.

What makes this hard to do:

You must overcome the tendency to react immediately to a disrespectful situation. That takes training, so you'll need to practice.

Many people truly believe you *should* not be so sensitive and *ought* to get past your sensitivity. But consider whether you want to dull the beautiful sensitivity you have and can use in your behalf in other kinds of situations. Instead, develop new ways to deal with disrespectful and harsh situations.

FINDING WAYS TO SIT STILL

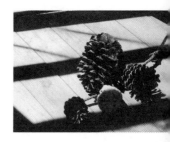

DO YOU FIND IT HARD, EVEN PAINFUL IF NOT IMPOSSIBLE, TO STAY STILL?

You're attending a gathering in which you don't play an active role, emotionally or physically. Though you want to be there, your body is rebelling at the need to be still. Even when you try to be still, you discover you're moving.

Why this happens:

■ Your physical activity level is high. It's just the way you're made. You're naturally much better off standing, walking, and moving about than sitting. You do these things well. You just don't sit quietly.

■ Some people are more expressive than others, so they may noticeably tap, thump, and fidget. Others are quieter and call less attention to their restlessness, but they still feel bad when required to be still.

■ Sitting for a length of time that is longer than your body's comfort limit leads to physical pain. You move to relieve the discomfort.

- You tend to learn and work better when some part of your body is moving.

- You're not moving in response to anyone else. You aren't doing it *to them*. But if another person doesn't have the same style as you do, he or she probably doesn't understand and may take what you do personally.

- Our culture seems to believe that "stillness is preferred to activity" in many situations. On the other hand, activity becomes an asset when applied to sports or being a "go-getter." So part of the issue to be dealt with has to do with assessing the situation in which you find your-self. Work with the situations that cause you trouble, but don't attempt to become a quiet person.

What not to do:

Don't let your high activity level control you and draw attention to you if you don't want it to.

What to do:

1. Do learn ways to accommodate your activity level so *you* are comfortable and so you don't bother others.

2. Acknowledge and accept your need for movement. (Hummingbirds don't apologize for being very active.) Be prepared ahead of time to avert problems caused by your activity level.

3. Whenever possible, put yourself in situations where you have freedom of movement. For example, if you're a salesperson, get a job in outside sales rather than one where you sit at a desk all day, tethered to a phone.

   If you go to the movies, choose a theater that has seats that are big enough and separate enough from the ones around you that your movement doesn't also move the person next to you. Better yet, find a theater that has seats that rock. Some of the newer ones have these, and they are truly made for those of us

Behaving Yourself

with bodies that like to move.

If you're giving a talk, use a lapel microphone that lets you move around rather than requiring you to stand behind a podium with a stationary microphone.

If you are in meetings, classes, or other gatherings where you fear you may bother someone and you tend to rapidly raise one or both of your heels or toes, you would do well to keep your feet out of sight, tucked under a table. That will reduce the visible distraction for others. You can also place your hands on your upper legs so you feel the result of the movement of your feet as they come off the floor. Or you can cut a deal with a close friend to reach over and place his or her hand on your knee. That will serve as a reminder to settle down.

4. Consider sitting near the back of the room so you can unobtrusively get up and lean against a doorjamb or counter when sitting becomes impossible. You may wish to walk around quietly or rock gently back and forth on your feet while you listen to someone speak.

5. Take something with you that you can "fiddle with." This will help you release pent-up tension. This can be a paper clip in your pocket, a plastic bead suspended between two knots on a leather thong, or any small object that you can fool with that does not make noise. Make a leather thong or use a piece of string with a bead strung between the two knotted ends. You can then silently slide the bead between the knots.

6. Take some kind of handwork to any meeting you have to attend. Feel free to tell the speaker that you listen better if you are doing something with your hands.

7. Draw pictures.

8. You may find that taking notes of

what is being said and done or recording your thoughts helps you not only sit still, but helps you pay attention to what's going on.

9. Learn a silent resistance exercise technique such as isometrics that releases tension and actually builds body strength at the same time.

10. When your legs are crossed, it's usually your foot that swings up and down. If you fear the swinging is disruptive to others, cross your ankles so your foot isn't loose for swinging. Then wiggle your toes inside your shoes to drain off your need to move.

11. Letting your toes dance inside of your shoes is a great way to discharge built-up energy. Notice if you hear (think or sense) tunes in your mind while moving your toes against the inside of your shoes. Or maybe you create rhythms, patterns, or number sequences with various toes as you lift and drop them inside your shoes.

12. With finger tapping, you will need to be especially careful that you don't have a hard object in your hand that will cause a sound. That can be very irritating to others. Try, instead, to depress your fingers on a tabletop, arm rest, or your own arm or leg. Again, follow rhythmic and musical patterns and count if you wish. You can do this without visibly moving your fingers.

13. Don't try to work longer than your "sitting span" will comfortably allow.

14. Have an office chair that rocks and swivels and gently rotate it while working, listening, or talking on the phone. Be sure to use a cordless phone.

15. When you're in a work situation, immediately look around for ways to escape. For example, use trips to the secretary's desk, drinking fountain,

and supply room as "sitting breaks." Let's say you're working at home on your computer. Use simple household chores as breaks. Turn on the garden hose. Turn it off. Put the laundry in. Take the laundry out. None of these will take much time, but they'll get you up and moving.

What makes this hard to do:

One of the hardest parts of keeping still is believing that *any* motion is wrong. Small, unobtrusive motions that relieve your stress and do not bother those around you are the answer.

View from the Cliff

QUIETING A NOISY MIND

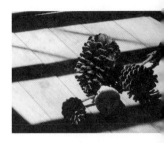

DO YOU HAVE A MIND THAT CHATTERS, THINKS, AND IS CONSTANTLY IMAGINING ALL SORT OF THINGS?

No matter what the time of day, your mind seems to be a mass of booming, buzzing, sometimes confusing thoughts. Often they tire you out, not to mention distract you from whatever you're trying to focus on. When you are tired and want to rest, your mind may not quit even at night.

Why this happens:

- As a sensitive person, you will notice and absorb large amounts of stimulation from your environment. Subjected to so much input, you will find your mind filling to capacity. Your sensitivity also extends to noticing what you feel emotionally and physically from your own body.

- If you have experienced trauma or difficult emotional experiences, you will likely have a large amount of post-traumatic images, sounds, and feelings as your mind tries to make sense of them and heal you.

- Without a way to drain off, organize, or release this input, it will tend to chaotically churn about in your mind.

- When you are excited by or even focused on a project, you will tend to stir up even more creative ideas as you see the many implications of each strand of your thinking. This happens when The True You has a predominantly analog style of brain construction that automatically networks and connects lots of details into patterns.

What not to do:

Neither allow this mental busy-ness to wear you out nor medicate it into stillness without working first with natural means to direct, utilize, and calm the flow.

What to do:

1. Gently search for quieter, less stimulating environments in which to place yourself while finding natural, healthy ways to soothe and calm your mind.

   You can begin to work on your environment first or you can begin to discover ways to calm your mind. Or you can do both simultaneously.

2. When you begin to work with your environment, assess the amount of stimulation in your environment. Spend a day or two noticing your surroundings. Pay attention to sounds, movements, reflections, colors, and textures. Utilize all your senses: sight, hearing, smell, taste, touch, and the gut-level feelings that pick up the emotional tone of your environment. You may be surprised to discover you are exposing yourself to a variety of feeling tones: tense, frenetic, angry, soothing, joyful, fearful, or a multitude of other emotional tones.

3. Analyze and evaluate each type of stimulus you receive. Consider ask-

ing yourself a series of questions.

"Is the sound around me noisy or soft sounding?"

"Is it pleasant or irritating?"

"Is there a lot of movement in my environment?"

"Is it predictable or unpredictable?"

"Do I find the movement pleasant or unpleasant?"

"Are the patterns I see busy, blended, rigid, geometrical?"

"Do I like or dislike the patterns that surround me?"

"Are there many or a few colors surrounding me?"

"Do the colors seem to clash or blend together?"

"Am I surrounded by my favorite colors?"

"Am I surrounded by any colors I dislike?"

"What are the textures to which I'm exposed?"

"Do I like them? Do they feel good?"

"Is the environment natural or manufactured?"

"Do I prefer to be inside or outside?"

"Do I prefer a rural or an urban environment?"

4. Note how many aspects of your environment please you.

5. If a lot displease you, what can you do about it? Ask yourself how much control you have over your surroundings. Immediately consider how you can make them more com-

patible. How can you calm down your environment or smooth it out so your mind is less stimulated? Many people are put on mental overload by working in the city. They find country living a necessity. Certain sounds bring calm to people. Some folks like the ongoing sound of the sea while others like the steady drum of traffic and city life. Find your own preferences and work to spend as much time as possible in the ones you like.

6. Consider using a tape recorder with earplugs through which you can listen to the sounds you like.

7. In seeking ways to calm your mind, try meditation. It is one of the most successful means to acquire mental calmness. This does not necessarily mean an "empty your mind" form of meditation. For active minds, this is not a realistic goal. Guided meditation often works well with busy-minded people. There are audio tapes and training programs available to assist you in finding what works best for you. Sample them until you find what works best for you.

8. Certain tones and sounds are soothing. In particular you may be drawn to the sounds of nature, such as live birds, especially cooing doves, running water, wind in trees, frogs croaking, and so on. On the other hand, you might feel calmed by totally different sounds. Rock and roll works for some people.

9. Mental visualization of pleasant scenes helps many folks meditate. If you have fond memories from childhood, pull these up into your mind's eye. Or create a fantasy scene or replicate one you've noticed in the movies or on TV.

10. Massage, polarity, and cranial-sacral therapy as well as other forms of bodywork utilized on a regular basis

can do wonders to relax your mind.

11. Activities such as gardening, long-distance running, and working on a potter's wheel, to name a few, calm some people. There are many activities from which to choose. Don't forget television.

12. Journaling and drawing pictures of your thoughts may also effectively remove them from your mind.

What makes this hard to do:

It can take time to make environmental changes. And it takes time to work with your own inner processes to find what's soothing for you. Sometimes major life changes are necessary if you are to find a fit for The True You, but the results can be extremely satisfying. Life is too short to continually expose yourself to environments that don't fit.

Taking the time to train your inner mind is worth every moment you put into it. It's ranked up there with good nutrition and physical fitness.

Caution: If you suffer from obsessive thinking in which the *same* thoughts repeat over and over and over in your mind, you would do well to consult a professional who treats this type of disturbance to your well-being.

TALKING LOTS AND LOTS

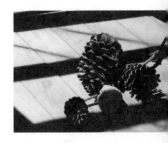

DO YOU TALK INCESSANTLY?

When you were a child, your teachers said what a chatterbox you were. They thought it was kind of cute. But you've begun to notice that people at work sometimes say, "I haven't time to listen" or "Get to the point." Even your spouse, who used to like your talkativeness, says, "Give it a rest." You wonder if your talking is becoming a problem.

Why this happens:

■ Just as some people are typically very physically active, some people are verbally active.

■ The amount of talking you do also depends on the environment in which you were raised. So if you were raised in a family whose members talk a lot, you are likely to feel comfortable talking, unless no one ever listened to you.

■ If people rarely listened to you, you may feel a need to talk a lot in order to be heard.

■ You may think you'd better share whatever is on your mind *right now*, or you fear you'll forget it.

- If you were not taught to listen as well as talk, you may not realize that you overtalk or "hog the stage," leaving no room for dialogue. That gets irritating to others.

- Different situations determine the amount of talking that is useful. A friendly off-hours conversation can go on for hours while on-the-job, bottom-line interchanges need to be succinct. A problem will arise if you don't distinguish between settings.

- Sometimes people talk endlessly in an attempt to talk someone into something. That is a power play.

- Sometimes people talk a lot for emotional reasons, trying to justify what they want or are doing. Feelings of inadequacy create this kind of talking behavior.

What not to do:

Do not ignore other people's reactions to you, but also know you deserve to be heard.

What to do:

1. Be in charge of the talking you do so that you are effectively heard, appreciated, and understood.

2. Notice if you're dominating conversations. Pay attention to how much the other person says. Notice whether the other person begins to form words, opens his mouth, or starts to say something as you talk over him in order to finish what you are thinking about.

3. If a person snickers and rolls her eyes while she's with you, ask what the nonverbal expression means. These are all signs that something is amiss. It may or may not be a response to your talking.

4. Make a note to stop talking right away when someone has something to say so you can learn to share con-

versation time. Even if you lose your train of thought, you are reaching for a more important goal—to learn to converse. In time, you will be able to both talk and listen without forgetting. (See Talking Off Track, p. 50.)

5. Before starting to talk, ask the other person, "How much time do you have to talk?" or "Are you on a deadline?" "Do you have time for a story or shall I save it for later?" If the person is short on time, get right to the point without explanations or stories.

6. Analyze your talking by asking some hard questions of yourself. "Do I press people to do things by verbally trying to convince them? Do I badger people into giving me what I want?" If so, give others the respect of accepting their negative responses with grace. Don't nag.

7. Check out how much you try to jus-tify to others your actions, your thoughts, and maybe your very existence. Though it feels bad to feel insecure, it's *your* job to learn to feel better about yourself, not theirs. So don't talk about it endlessly to everyone with whom you come in contact.

8. Assume that anyone you're doing business with accepts you and your skill level. See yourself as a capable person. (If you can't pull this off on your own, check in with a counselor to help you.)

9. If you've gotten yourself into a situation where someone doesn't value you and after talking with the person you still do not feel appreciated, consider finding a more compatible job or personal fit.

10. You may have been trained growing up that you can get your needs met by talking someone else to exhaustion. Or you may try to override

what another person wants by wearing him or her down. These are power plays and do not belong in mutually respectful relationships. Stop it!

What makes this hard to do:

Verbal habits and brain construction can add up to a lot of talking. You'll need to sort out how much of your talking is habit and how much is innate. Then commit to owning up to what you can change. You may never be a quiet person, but you can rein yourself in enough to be an enjoyable, if not delightful, person to be around.

Caution: Incessant talking that does not yield to your conscious attempts to control it may be due to an imbalance in your brain chemistry that is called *obsessive talking.* If this is the case, you may be unable to control your talking without medical help. This is rare, however.

BLURTING THINGS OUT

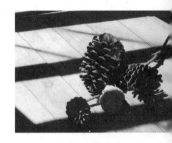

DO YOU SAY THINGS WITHOUT THINKING?

When you recently went to visit your grandmother, she took you to her reading group and to your dismay, you embarrassed her and yourself. Someone asked if you were married and without thinking about where you were, you said, "Well not exactly, but we've been living together for a couple of years."

You wonder why you say such things. Only a few days earlier, your boss asked you if you'd buy some of the candy his daughter was selling for a money raiser. In response you blurted out, "Yuk, that candy tastes like tar." What in the world were you thinking? You know better than to compromise your job by ignoring office politics.

Besides airing your preferences at inopportune times, you have a bad habit of saying what you think. For example, your best friend came by with a new dress and haircut and out of your mouth pops, "Where'd you get that thing?" Then as if that wasn't bad enough, you added, before you noticed the horrified look on her face, "Who scalped you?" It's a good thing you've known each other for years or you'd have one less friend. But you hate it when you hurt anyone's feelings. That's not your intent.

Why this happens:

- The way you're made benefits you *and* causes trouble. You are a keen observer, have a strong personality, and are very emotional. You also are likely to speak before you think. It's all part of your brainstyle.

- The more expressively dramatic and verbally active you are, the more you will tend to show your feelings and act upon them.

- But some of your behavior is the result of having been reinforced, even in a negative way, for your outbursts. And the reinforcement has probably been going on for a long time. Or maybe you've been trying to change someone's behavior by telling them what to do.

- You undoubtedly have an expressive nature, but if you haven't found appropriate channels for your expression, the inner need to discharge your talents will override your social judgment.

- As you have gotten older, part of your identity is tied as much to what you do wrong as what you do right. If you were not able to get things right early on, you, like all people, will tend to automatically go to the opposite extreme of being the most outrageous person you can be.

What not to do:

Do not continue to act in a way that doesn't serve you.

What to do:

1. Learn to use your strong energy and skillful verbal potential in ways that clearly express who you are and get you self-esteem-enhancing attention.

2. First list your observational skills.

Behaving Yourself

Are you quick to size up a situation? Do you tend to see the truth under surface charades?

3. List your expressive skills. Are you good with words? Expressions? Gestures? Are you funny? Quick witted? Do people find you entertaining? Are you a good storyteller?

4. Ask yourself if you have a strong belief system. Do you stick with it when you are in the minority, like when you were with your grandmother and were the only one who was okay about living with someone to whom you aren't married?

5. Once you've finished an assessment of your assets, look at your inner feelings of self-confidence and self-esteem. Do you find a difference between your talents and your inner feelings? If so, the discrepancy probably comes because you've developed your skills as an adult, but your feelings stem from when you were young and much more susceptible to others' judgments.

6. Ask yourself whether you've been continually reinforced, positively or negatively, for blurting out things that amaze others and end up embarrassing you. Or have you been trying to fix another person's problem? Has there been a particular person in your life who has made a big deal of your blurting things out?

7. When you're ready, have a mental dialogue with that person, saying, "I know you haven't understood or been able to respond constructively to me. I'm now taking over the job of being in charge of my behavior, including my mouth. I appreciate what you've tried to do, and I forgive both of us for what didn't work. Neither of us understood that I could eventually learn to effectively take charge of myself, including my

mouth, and let you take charge of yourself."

8. Now think and feel about how you want to be. Ask yourself how you would like to express yourself. In what settings? Would you like to be dramatic? Then consider taking up theater arts work, improvisational activities, or speaking. If you'd like to speak out on behalf of a social issue, do so. Become verbal for a cause. Maybe you have an interest in motivating others. You could even become a radio personality, teacher, or counselor. But whatever direction you take, know that the very mouth that has gotten you in trouble can be used for constructive purposes now.

9. Once you've opened the door for effective self-expression, you can begin to work on keeping your mouth shut when you choose. Look at listening as a skill that will provide you with information.

10. Store what you hear for later use. Make notes as soon as possible about what you censored. These will provide great fodder for future speaking, writing, and storytelling.

11. Once you've begun to learn to be quiet and listen, assess situations in which you find yourself. Ask what others need. What is their world-view? What do they value? How much can they handle?

12. Decide if you want to fit into their worldview for the time being or be a renegade. There are times and places for each choice.

13. You now have the tools to say what you wish when you want to speak. Congratulate yourself. You've become an expressive person who can also listen and control yourself when you choose.

What makes this hard to do:

If you have a long history of seeing yourself as an impulsive speaker, you are likely to feel helpless about changing. Though you may feel as if you face a daunting task, you can reshape your talking one step at a time.

TAKING ON TOO MUCH

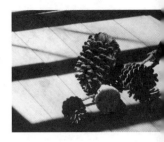

DO YOU GET YOURSELF IN OVER YOUR HEAD BY OVERCOMMITTING?

You've gone and done it again! You said, "I'll do it." You volunteered to take on a project at the very time you are already on overload with too much to do. It's getting toward the end of the school year, for example, and not only are you loaded with teaching duties, but you coach, are planning to help out a friend for the summer, and you've already promised your family you'll do a lot of camping and special trips.

As if that's not enough, you opened your mouth when your church asked for someone to take an exchange student for next year. And he will be arriving early *this summer.*

You're always doing that, taking on more than any one human can hope to accomplish. To be honest, though, you usually pull everything off, but at what cost? You worry that maybe it's not good for your kids, not to mention your spouse and your health.

Why this happens:

■ First of all, you undoubtedly have an enormously high level of physical energy. That simply means that you're constructed in a way that supports your engaging in many tasks without collapsing.

- The way your brain is constructed lends itself to multitasking.

- Add in your personality style that makes you a "helper type"—one who feels the need to respond to other people's needs—and you'll find it hard to turn requests down.

- You are likely to be sensitive, which is part of the reason you are aware of others' needs. If you're also kinesthenic, another aspect of that sensitivity means you'll want *to do something to fix* the discomfort created by a need you see. So you act *to fix* whatever presents itself as much for yourself as for the other person.

- Taking on so many things at once probably also means you have a brainstyle that predisposes you to become totally immersed in each thing you're doing as if it is the only thing you're doing. You tend to forget there are several of these "total immersion" activities going on at the same time. While you're engaged in one activity, it is the whole world to you. It's easy to forget when you are being asked to do something that you already said yes to a lot of other things.

- Occasionally, people do lots and lots in order to *prove* their worthiness. Though this explanation is often given, it is frequently not the real reason for overcommitting. More often there's nothing pathological about taking on a lot. It's more likely the way you perceive and experience your life events as they are shaped by your brainstyle.

What not to do:

Do not think there is something *wrong* with you because you do a lot, but also don't let yourself get so carried away that you shortchange the special people in your life, including yourself.

What to do:

1. Put yourself in control of what you choose to do so you can get quality as well as quantity out of life.

2. Identify the different commitments, obligations, and projects in which you're currently engaged. You can either do this exercise mentally or write out your response on paper. You might list family, paying job, hobby, neighbors, and volunteer work.

3. If you choose to write down your list, put the name for each project, commitment, or obligation on a separate sheet of paper.

4. Rank the categories in order of importance to you and place the papers in that order.

5. Divide the various tasks that you are doing according to the categories you've selected. You may find that you have two different hobbies, two ways you earn money, one family obligation (with another pending), two neighbors you help, and three community projects.

6. Write the individual projects under the headings you've already created. Each sheet will have the name of the category at the top. Under it you will list the different projects by name. One sheet might read *Neighbors* at the top. Under it you would write: Ken and Joe.

7. Then step back, having laid the papers out in front of you. Look at them for a few seconds.

8. Then shut your eyes and breathe deeply. Ask yourself, "What's really important to me?" You may want to get away by yourself to sort out your feelings about this question.

9. Once you've become clear about your priorities at this time, not for the rest of your life, but for now, again look at the papers. Reassess the commitments you have made. Follow through on the ones you've said you will do, but don't add any more until you work out a limit for how much you realistically can do.

10. Remain clear about your priorities, and review them if you need to. Now decide how many commitments you want under each category. Let's say your main categories are:

Categories	Commitments
Family	1
Paying Job	2
Hobbies	2
Neighbors	2
Community Projects	3

Put the number of commitments you have after each category. Ask yourself, "Am I overloaded in any of the categories?" "Do I need to elimi-nate something?" "Do I need to eliminate a category?"

If you are overloaded, don't take on any more until you have finished what you've started.

11. The number of commitments is less important than how you feel about what you are doing. Psychologically and physically you'll feel more drained by some events and projects than others. Your emotional reactions will tell you which to keep and what to change. Deep inside, you know when you need to eliminate.

Listen! You'll hear warning signs in your head that tell you to slow down. Maybe you hear, "I really shouldn't say I'll do it." "My wife will kill me for this." Maybe you feel your stomach twist. Or perhaps you feel guilty for taking on another task. These are all signs that you are going too far.

12. Ask yourself whether you fear that you'll never be able to do something

you want to do if you say no now. This is a frequent reason people overload. This can be a strong fear, but it's unfounded. You can almost always reconnect with a desire later on. You don't have to do everything now.

13. Learn to say no. You need to get in the habit of saying no. To buy time, never make your decisions immediately. Say, "Let me think about this, and I'll get back to you tomorrow." By doing this, you're forming a habit, one that will stand you in good stead in many ways throughout your life.

14. Having bought time, you can review your commitments. Check to see if you have room for an additional task in the category in which it fits.

15. Acquire a "commitment buddy." This is someone who will listen to you talk through the potential addition of something to your schedule. This person won't make the decision for you, but will remind you that you tend to overload and will help you be strong in saying no.

16. When you tell someone no but would like to keep the door open for the future, you can say, "I can't let myself take this on now, but I'd like to consider it later."

17. People will respect you for this approach. Your family will appreciate your willingness to spend time with them, and you will be in control of your life.

What makes this hard to do:

Probably the hardest part of working on overcommitment is the feeling you'll miss out on something. Always promise yourself that you'll get back to whatever you're putting aside. Things of importance will always hang around, and you can nurture them into reality whenever you wish.

Behaving Yourself

ATTENDING TO R & R

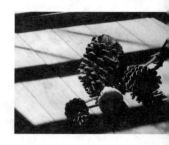

IS IT HARD FOR YOU TO FIND THE TIME FOR REST AND RELAXATION (R & R)?

You work hard. After all, you are a high-energy person. And you like challenges. You've known you ought to relax some of the time, but you never seem to get around to it. Besides, you really like being busy. If you're completely honest, you may have to admit that the few times you've taken time off, you've not had a very good time. You either slept all the time, drank too much, or got restless and bored after a day.

Why this happens:

■ Being a naturally active person, you know more about doing things than not doing things. Doing little or nothing may seem foreign to you.

■ When your main focus of attention is on work and family, you undoubtedly have a full schedule. To make time for R & R takes planning. And if that's not your strong suit, you could easily skip much needed break time.

■ If you don't plan regularly for R & R, you are likely to put it off until you're exhausted. Then is not the best time to find pleasant, fun things to do. For one thing, you have to catch up from your exhaustion before you can enjoy yourself.

■ You may also remember that there were too many times growing up when you could not be as active as you liked. So being inactive feels bad now. Such painful memories can lead to doing whatever you can to dull that pain, including drinking, using drugs, running away—things like that.

What not to do:

Do not ignore your need for R & R or wait until you're exhausted to do something about it.

What to do:

1. Plan R & R time into your life in a form that easily fits you and your lifestyle and brainstyle.

2. To find the right way for you, you'll need to notice whether you do things better if they are formally scheduled into your calendar or are better left to an inner sense of when you need R & R.

    Notice if you can tune into your body's needs. Some people can. Others can't. If you can, note whether you have the freedom to manage your own schedule. If you're a self-employed person who works at home, your time may well be under your control. Then you can work sixteen hours one day and skip working the next.

    If, however, you have outside commitments that leave little flexibility in your schedule, you'll probably need to set a specific time aside on a regular basis.

3. Next decide if you prefer getting your R & R regularly, like exercising three times a week, or intermittently, like taking a long weekend every couple of months or after you finish

a big project. Do you prefer a lot of little breaks or a few longer ones?

4. Note the difference between rest and recreation. Doing something different from what you normally do, even if it's active, can be as rehabilitating as sleeping or doing nothing.

5. If you're having trouble keeping on track with your R & R, check to see if what you're doing fits you. Going to a gym makes some people feel great, while others feel awful as they pick up all kinds of excess energy from the environment. One person will love golf, or running, or holing up for a weekend with a stack of videos, while another will hate it. Some people's idea of R & R is to fly to Vegas, while another wants to wander in the woods alone. Don't pay attention to what others say you *ought* to do. Do whatever you want as long as it's not illegal or harmful to your health or another person. Disregard anyone who doesn't understand the choices you make.

6. Just as cross training helps keep some athletes' motivation high, so does doing a variety of activities work better for some people. Others like getting into a routine of doing the same thing all the time.

What makes this hard to do:

Friends and relatives may have their own ideas about what R & R ought to look like. Often they make suggestions and say, "You ought to go do. . . ." They are really saying, "*I* like to do such and such" and so assume that you will like it too. Be kind. Say, "Thank you." And don't succumb to their influence if it doesn't fit you.

DEALING WITH DRUG OR ALCOHOL USAGE

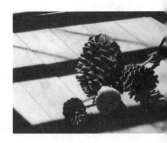

DO YOU WONDER WHETHER YOUR DRUG AND ALCOHOL TREATMENT JOURNEY IS IDENTICAL TO EVERYBODY ELSE'S?

A few months ago a relative sat you down and asked you to go to AA (Alcoholics Anonymous) with him. Your job had been very stressful lately, with more and more paperwork and details to cope with—paperwork and details that you hate. You didn't seem to be able to get ahead. Your spouse had been after you to get things cleaned up at home, and the kids were bouncing off the walls. You felt incredibly stressed.

You began to take a drink after work and found it made you feel better. A friend introduced you to "pot" and it helped relieve you from the stress of your job.

With your relative urging and supporting you, you started to attend AA. You quit drinking and learned a lot. But you still felt really stressed at work and at home. Your kids were doing poorly in school. Your home life was chaos, trying to get your kids to do their homework while you struggle with the housework. Meals, shopping, and the hundred million little jobs never seemed to get done on time.

At a school conference you began to learn about your kids' particular type of brain construction—one that does not lend itself to working with details and paperwork. You recognized yourself in them. You were just like them when you were in school. You still are. No wonder you feel so stressed out all the time. You also have discovered how sensitive you all are and how stress impacts you.

You've been going to classes to help your kids. And you're learning a lot about organizing in ways that fit you, too. You've learned that you are in the worst kind of job possible for The True You. Your immediate life has gotten easier and you've begun looking into other kinds of work that will fit you better. (See Finding Jobs That Fit, p. 243.) With these changes, you rarely feel down anymore. You see hope for all of you. You've given pot up, and you don't really care anymore if you have a drink.

You've begun to wonder whether your drug and alcohol journey is different from some of the other people in your AA program.

Why this happens:

- If you have been chronically under stress, pressured for as long as you can remember to do things that aren't a good fit for the way you're made, you are going to seek relief. Alcohol and "pot" are two of the more accessible ways to do that and are two typical drugs of choice by people with sensitive natures who find it hard to deal with situations that don't fit their brainstyle.

- Because of a lack of understanding of brain diversity, many people experience undue tension, anxiety, and depression daily. If you're like this, the stress disappears quickly when you learn ways to live day by day that fit your natural self.

- Drugs and alcohol medicate the secondary symptoms that result from living in a society that does not understand and hinders the expression of your natural brainstyle.

■ Twelve-step programs are designed for people with addictive personalities who need to continually work with their addictive tendencies. Or they help people who are suffering emotional and chronic pain from wounding at an earlier time.

Participants benefit from the support of others who have been down the road ahead of them. A constitutional addict does not lose the desire for drugs or alcohol by understanding brain construction or finding environments that fit. A psychologically wounded person doesn't lose the desire for drugs or alcohol by changing his or her environmental fit.

■ If you're medicating yourself to relieve stress created by a misfitting environment, and you're not constitutionally addictive, you will follow a different path to recovery. With information, environmental management, and the acquisition of skills that help you live according to your natural bent, you are likely to leave problems with chemical dependency behind.

What not to do:

Do not assume that everyone who uses drugs or drinks too much is chemically dependent for life. And do not use brain diversity as an excuse to indulge.

What to do:

1. Immediately cease drinking and using drugs and learn about the management of your particular style of brain construction.

2. Begin attending an AA or NA (Narcotics Anonymous) support group and learn the principles of a twelve-step program. Work your program.

3. Talk to people who have a similar brain construction to yours. Learn what they do to live naturally in a society that doesn't readily fit their particular style.

4. Learn what to do to relieve stress in your life. Learn about managing daily living at work and at home. Build a repertoire of skills that reflects your brainstyle.

5. Read about creative and successful people with a brain construction similar to yours.

6. Learn meditation techniques and ways to get R & R. (See Attending to R & R, p. 148.)

7. Check the career/job part of your life. Ask yourself, "Does it fit me? Am I feeling productive? Am I being myself, doing what I love to do? Am I glad, most of the time, to get up in the morning because I am pleased with my agenda for the day?"

8. If your answer is no to many of these questions, then immediately begin to restructure your work life. Consider engaging in career counseling that factors in brain diversity so you look at jobs that will fit you. Then make moves to change so you are in alignment with your potential and able to use it more fully and satisfactorily.

9. Next, check your personal life. Be sure that you are in a mutually respectful relationship—one in which you and your partner work as a team. You each need to focus on one another's diversity and your respective assets, not your liabilities.

10. Learn about diversity of brain construction in relation to household chores, entertainment, sex, and communication.

11. Apply what you learn by looking at the world through your partner's eyes. This is hard, but do the best you can. It takes time and lots of

talking, not arguing and not necessarily problem-solving, but sharing of perceptions with the emphasis on understanding and appreciating each other. Then, creatively find ways to meet both sets of needs.

12. As you attend a twelve-step program and come into alignment with your natural self, become aware of how similar and different you are to those around you.

13. Be aware of how much or little you continue to struggle with a desire for alcohol or drugs.

14. Consider whether you were responding to a lack of awareness of what The True You needed to be effective and at peace. If you were trying to reduce the stress of an ill-fitting environment, put emphasis on being sure you honor your brainstyle and true nature. As a result, you may find you have no need for alcohol or drugs.

What makes this hard to do:

Twelve-step programs have made an enormous contribution to all people who have addictions that rule their lives. Yet not everyone who becomes involved with alcohol and drugs requires ongoing dependency on the group for the rest of their lives.

This can be a scary thought for anyone who has struggled with chemical use. You and those around you will know whether you need continuous support of this type once you've honored your true self.

GETTING "HIGH"

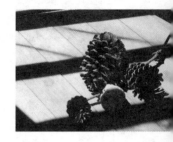

HAVE YOU GOTTEN INTO DIFFICULTY BECAUSE OF WANTING THE "HIGH" THAT COMES FROM THINGS YOU DO?

Fast driving, adventure, and new challenges all give you a high, whether it's learning to fly, outmaneuvering a competitor, or gambling on a high-stakes game. You really love the feeling you get when you nail a win or meet a challenge. You may have noticed the feeling of letdown when you don't get your run in or haven't had sex for a time. You manage, but you feel depressed.

Why this happens:

■ You are likely to be an incredibly sensitive person who feels everything acutely. That means you can get devastatingly hurt and joyously happy.

■ You live by your feelings more than your thinking. That's just how you are. Feelings provide you with information. You grow from them and you express through them.

■ If you have a high energy level to boot, physically, mentally, or verbally, you will also tend to have a high level of volatile feelings.

- If you are kinesthenic, you will tend to act out your feelings.

- One thing that makes some people feel good is doing something exciting. So you begin with the excitement that comes with doing something that has a risk or pushes the limits. You feel great as a result. You express your great feelings by acting on them. Then you get even more excited. Thus a cycle of excitement reinforces itself, increasing your good feelings—and that's very psychologically addictive.

- Moderation is lost in the cycle of excitement. Your behavior can take on an addictive tone as you seek more and more excitement.

- Untrained in the rhythm of your brain construction, you have little hope of finding a moderate way to handle the enormity of feelings and stimulation by which you live.

- In addition, every time you feel down, bored, or stressed, you are likely to recall how good you felt when you were doing something exciting that made you feel high. The temptation becomes strong to repeat an activity that brought you the good feeling previously, so off you go, taking a risk to make yourself feel better.

What not to do:

Do not let your feelings run rampant, and do not make promises that you'll "never seek excitement again."

What to do:

1. Seek outlets to achieve a "high" that do not get you into trouble while you are working on building your skills to achieve moderation.

2. Determine if you have a tendency to

overdo and overindulge in activities that give a high. To do this, ask yourself some questions.

"Do I overdo things?" Make a list of these things, starting with when you were a kid.

"Was I often told that I didn't know when to stop?" Who said this? In retrospect, was the person right even if you hate to admit it?

"Do I smirk or feel like a 'little dickens' who is getting away with something when I engage in an activity that excites me?"

"Do I feel as if I *have to* reach a 'high' either for relief or pleasure?

"What price have I had to pay for my overindulgence?" Be strictly honest here. List everything from scoldings as a child to confinement as an adult. What about loss of family, friends, or jobs? List little things as well as big losses.

"Am I tempted to keep on doing some things that give me a high even though I have made other commitments?"

"Can I walk away from something exciting without suffering?"

"When I get going on something that charges my emotions, can I let go of it for a time, knowing I can return to it at a later date?"

3. Look at your answers and get a sense of how stressful it is for you to move in and out of activities that excite you.

4. Become not only aware of your feelings and needs but be aware of their effect in relation to another person. Practice communicating your truth.

5. Begin to get familiar with the sensitivity that resides within you rather than immediately covering it with some form of activity that's accompanied by the enticing feeling a high brings.

6. Learn to protect and express your sensitivity in other ways than covering it with a "high" feeling. (See the sections on temper control, beginning on p. 109.)

7. Once you're clear on whether or not you have a problem being addicted to a "high," commit to yourself that you will find ways to experience good feelings, "highs," that won't hurt you or others.

8. Open new doorways through which your passionate nature can flow. Enjoy the many ways you can reach a high. The trick is to find things to do that are exciting *and* won't get you into trouble. They will need to have some risk. You can always become an adventure writer and travel to the source of your stories for information, or you can work abroad. There's mountaineering, rock climbing, acrobatic flying, race-car driving, deep-sea diving, and white-water rafting. Don't forget the whole arena of emergency service work: fire fighting, EMT, and paramedic services as well as undercover police work. There's the thrill of participating in organized sports, both individual and team. These are just a few of the exciting outlets that include risk and excitement as part of the reward of participation. All of these activities can be used as income producers as well as entertainment.

For more sedentary people, mental activities such as playing the stock market and becoming involved in games that have risk and excitement can be of interest. Improvisational theater, stand-up comedy, talk radio, and investigative reporting are still more options.

The main issue is to find a way to experience adventure and a "high" without compromising yourself, hurting others, or breaking the law.

9. Don't bother to make promises that things will be different next time— that you will settle down. They're unrealistic, even though you desire to be more moderate at the time you say it.

10. Be sure you have a strong support network of like-minded people. Use them liberally. This will include people who are successfully living a life that is full of excitement.

11. Be sure that if you are in an intimate relationship with someone who isn't constructed the way you are that you explain what you need. On the one hand, a supportive person can enjoy your pleasure and encourage you. On the other hand, you can give the person permission to raise an eyebrow at you, if you begin to fool

yourself or push reasonable limits too far.

12. But be cautious if you are constantly scolded for "how you are." You must simply "own" your own nature, holding up your end of being responsible for your activities. But don't let yourself be "tethered" to a traditional lifestyle that sucks you dry. If you do, you will tend to begin to sneak around and are more likely to get into some big trouble because you are not openly adjusting for your needs.

What makes this hard to do:

Only you can ultimately be responsible for control of yourself despite the intensity of the urges within you. You must know when and how to ask for help. You must be responsible for when you get off track and protect yourself from your innate tendency to seek a high that gets out of control. You must stand by your true self and not try to be anything you are not. You can do it!

OVERDOING ACTIVITIES

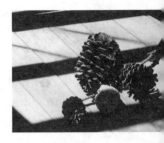

IF YOU LIKE SOMETHING, DO YOU USUALLY FIND YOURSELF DOING IT IN EXCESS?

You recently became interested in a new hobby and decided to take an evening class in it. Now a few months later, your spouse is complaining that you're never home and your kids have given up trying to get you to spend time with them. You suppose it's because your one-night class turned into a seven-day-a-week activity.

You love it. It makes you feel calm and totally quiets your mind. But you have to admit that almost anything you like ends up consuming you. Last year it was something else. Before that, yet one more interesting hobby absorbed you. It's not that you don't want to be at home. You really don't care whether you do the activity at home or away from home. It's just that once you start something, you become totally absorbed in it until your family complains so much that you have to give it up altogether.

Why this happens:

■ You are likely to be a person who

tends to be able to do only one thing at a time. It's the way your brain works, sort of like you have an "On-Off Switch" without a dimmer control to modulate the light. As a result you tend to become absorbed in whatever you are doing to the exclusion of all else.

- Add to this your tendency to be someone who experiences life primarily through your sensitive feelings.

- You are likely to emotionally flood— be flooded with feelings and stimulation—so that you will experience an onslaught of emotion. (See Feeling Overwhelmed, p. 186.) As a result, when something feels good, it feels "fantastically" good.

- Also, if you are a person who does not readily break big projects into small pieces, you may have difficulty finding your way step by step through anything you try to do. Instead, you dive in headfirst and grab onto whatever feels good. You cling to that until something else very important gets your attention.

- So here you are: a sensitive, emotionally porous person without defined limits who has difficulty moving from one step to another. You feel everything intensely and are already probably bruised by a world that is tough on people constructed like you. It's no wonder you revel in any good feeling that comes your way.

What not to do:

Do not helplessly succumb to your behavior, overlooking others' needs and failing to live a responsible life.

What to do:

1. Find avenues to use your intensity constructively while paying attention to the important people in your life and taking responsibility for your daily living.

2. Realize that you have a natural tendency to focus exclusively on one thing at a time. Because this can seduce you to lose yourself in an activity, you are likely to lose track of time. But when you do lose track of time, you lose track of your life. You will need to take steps to be sure that is how you want to live your life.

3. Revisit your value system. Ask yourself, "How do I want to live my life? How do I want to use my time?"

4. Make an assessment of your spiritual beliefs about *how* you choose to spend your time on earth.

5. Once you've begun to learn about what you want and how you want to live, reinforce your choices by enriching your spiritual life. Spiritual and religious paths assist in helping us use our time wisely when we tend toward being compulsive. They help us connect with a structure that is "bigger" and more powerful than our humanness. They will help you control your tendency to overindulge.

   Spirituality and religion also have an emotional component that you need. As a result, they provide structure *in the context* of feeling, which is an essential element to people with the style of brain construction that you have.

6. Next, turn to your family and those about whom you care. Note their complaints.

7. Ask yourself, "Do I attempt to listen to the needs of those with whom I have a relationship? Am I so focused on something that I don't hear what others say?"

8. Tell your companion what you've been thinking. And tell the person that you want to change. After all, you don't want to ignore someone you care about.

9. Then think about the time that you'd like to spend with your family. Think about things as simple as eating dinner together, rocking the baby to sleep, doing chores, going on a date with your spouse, or helping the kids do homework or playing catch in the backyard. You don't need to commit to all of these things all the time. But start thinking about them and how much time you'd like to spend on some of them every week.

10. Ask your partner to also think about what he or she would like to have in the way of involvement from you.

11. Talk together, noting the times you both desire to make available for joint activities. Negotiate differences.

12. Next, you'll need some way to keep track of your time. If you're already using a day scheduler for work, you may want to continue to use it at home. Plot in time for your family

and for any interest you wish to enjoy. This may seem impersonal and even cold, but remember you're doing it to help you live out your intent.

13. Ask yourself, "Do I become enabled to maintain my intense interest in something at the expense of being irresponsible to others on the job or in my family?" "Do others let me get away with shirking chores and jobs for which I need to be responsible?"

14. If you are being enabled to over-focus, it's up to you to take responsibility to stop it. *You* must commit to change the pattern of being out of control.

15. Once you've gotten straight with yourself, turn to your enabler and share your new understanding. Own up to the fact that you've not been listening or committed to helping to fulfill his or her needs. Acknowledge

you've not been taking on joint responsibilities. Say you are now aware and planning to change. Ask the person to stop enabling you.

16. Become specific. For example, if you pursue your activity past dinner time, the family is to go ahead and eat. If you're still not present when dinner is over, the food is to be put away and you're on your own. And you don't get to leave your dirty dishes in the sink after you finally eat.

17. You may need to rework your family budget if your activity is using a disproportionate amount of money. It's up to you to suggest making a new budget. If you "let your spouse come up with the idea," then it's like a parent putting a kid *on* a budget. You're not a kid.

    Basically figure out how much of your joint income is for necessities. This means housing, utilities, auto expenses, clothing, etc. It doesn't mean an extravagant car or designer clothes. Those would be paid for from discretionary income. If you can agree on how much to set aside for the future, such as income to invest, to put in your kid's school fund, or to put in a retirement fund, you're ready for the next step.

    Next, divide in half whatever is left over from the necessities and the savings for future expenses. This money each of you can do with as you wish. If you choose to use all of your discretionary income for one activity, that's your business. But don't expect your spouse to cover for you when there's an opportunity to do something together that might be fun.

    If you can't agree (even with counseling) on the amount of money to be set aside for the future, you might divide the income after necessities one of the following ways: You can divide what's left into equal portions for each family member, including children. Theirs can go into their school fund or an investment to be used if something happens to you.

As a result, your partner may be investing for the future while you may not. The problem with this, of course, is that you won't be ready for the future when it comes. That time may seem far off, or you figure you'll have enough to make it up later. But it will put enormous pressure on your partner to turn his or her back on you if you are ever in need at a later date. This lack of responsibility for the future can put a terrible strain on a relationship. Remember, you must be responsible in the future for the choices you make now.

There is only one way to resolve monetary imbalances in a family because of one person spending exorbitant amounts of money on an activity: legally become separate.

No matter how you handle money

issues, it behooves you to face them squarely now.

18. Begin to help others who are like you to become aware of how you are constructed and what you're doing to help yourself. Show them how you are balancing a tendency to focus on one thing at a time while staying involved with your family and spending your time so it is thoughtfully under your control. You will be reinforced in your mastery by helping others.

What makes this hard to do:

Most people in today's world are looking for a magic cure—the "pill" or intervention that will change them. Instead, you must accept how you are constructed and live in the process of using your traits positively and responsibly.

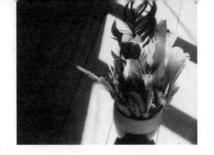

PART FOUR

Using and Protecting Your Sensitivity

Healing is a matter of time, but it is sometimes also a matter of opportunity.

HIPPOCRATES

460–377 B.C.

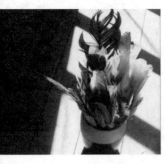

As with so many of our attributes that are affected by our style of brain construction, our physical and emotional sensitivity has an up side and a down side. The True You benefits from its level of sensitivity by reflecting compassion, empathy, keen observational skills, and the ability to creatively express beyond the lines of orthodox definitions. Functioning outside the boundaries of traditional thinking depends upon the flexibility and responsiveness of your natural limits—limits shaped by your creative style of brain construction.

But The Wounded You will have been hurt because of your sensitivity as you failed to effectively protect yourself from unwanted intrusions: actions, thoughts, and feelings. To be told "Don't be so sensitive" has been useless. You know you are as sensitive as your brainstyle dictates, not more and not less.

This section of View from the Cliff *will help you honor your sensitivity so you can make quality use of it while simultaneously learning how to protect your vulnerability. The Accommodating You will learn many skills to protect your sensitivity while allowing you to stay active in a potentially hurtful environment. As a result, you will be able to utilize The True You to its maximum potential as you protect The Wounded You from further hurt.*

CATCHING ANOTHER'S FEELINGS

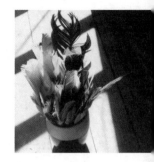

ARE YOU AN EMOTIONALLY SENSITIVE PERSON WHOSE MOODS SHIFT EASILY?

You're happily going about your business of the day. All of sudden, your mood shifts, dramatically. You feel depressed, really in the pits, and nothing happened to change it. All you did was talk to your friend at lunch. You didn't talk about anything upsetting. You worry that you may have an emotional *disorder*.

Why this happens:

■ If you get around someone who is experiencing feelings that he or she is not aware of or isn't dealing with and your emotional boundaries are thin, you are likely to begin to take on that person's feeling. You "catch their feelings," much as you would catch someone's cold, only this is on an emotional level. This happens because your emotional boundaries are porous and another's feelings of anger, sadness, anxiety, etc., simply flow into you.

- Let's say you ask someone how they are and the response is, "I'm fine." But you get a funny feeling that they're not fine. You are at high risk to feel whatever that person is feeling but is not aware of or not acknowledging underneath the "I'm fine" comment. This is your empathy at work as you experience what he or she is not expressing.

- The reasons for a mood shift often go unnoticed by those insensitive to them.

- Sometimes mood shifts happen when something you see, hear, or otherwise sense reminds you of a past experience. You recognize the feeling attached to that experience, and it can quickly and strongly change your emotions.

What not to do:

Don't automatically think there is something wrong with you. And do not assume your mood shifted for no reason.

What to do:

1. Realize that there are *real*, tangible reasons for any mood shift you experience, even if they are not readily apparent to outside observers. You may even fail to notice the source of a mood shift because you've been taught that "You just have mood shifts because your chemistry is off."

2. Pay attention to what you were doing and thinking right before your mood changed. Ask yourself, "Who was I with? Who was I around, even at a distance? What's happening here? What was I feeling? What was I thinking?" A mood shift can be caught from outside of you or stimulated by an inner thought.

3. As you ask the questions, note the images that go through your mind, or bits of conversation that play in your head or feelings that you get in

your body. It may take a little doing to heighten your awareness, but you will discover that your memory banks stored the trigger for your mood shift. All you have to do is recoup the memory. And it may come forth in a picture, word phrase, or sensation.

4. Believe in what you think, feel, and see.

5. If it is someone you know, check and see if you often feel a certain way around the person.

6. If the way you are feeling is not a way you'd like to continue to feel, it's important to separate yourself from the other person's feelings.

7. Keeping the other person in mind, you can say to yourself, "I pull my identification out of the situation." Or you may say, "I do not identify with so and so's feelings."

8. Visualize yourself breaking the emotional connection that attaches you to that person's feelings as if you are cutting cords that tie you together.

9. Check to see if you begin to feel better within minutes.

10. Arm yourself emotionally with a nonporous coating if you have to be around the person repeatedly. This could be visualized as a coat of armor, distance, or a fabric that emotions can't penetrate.

11. Give yourself permission to stay distant from that person. Or think of your hearts or minds connecting without a residue of unacknowledged feelings attached.

What makes this hard to do:

Being susceptible to others' feelings and outer influences because of your porous emotional boundaries is a fairly new idea in this culture. Therefore, you may not find much understanding or support in what you're doing and how you're feeling. Even those you love may think there is something wrong with you. Often professionals will label you with an emotional problem that is called "biochemical," when really you are simply reflecting the effects of emotional energy that is coming your way unnoticed.

BEING SUGGESTIBLE

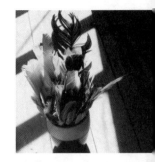

DO YOU CATCH THE MOOD OF THE GROUP IN WHICH YOU FIND YOURSELF, SOMETIMES TO YOUR DISADVANTAGE?

You enter a room and notice that your mood quickly changes depending upon the mood of the group. If the tone is somber, you begin feeling down, but if there are high spirits, you become almost manic. Sometimes you're so influenced by the group that you do things you wouldn't do if you were by yourself.

Why this happens:

- Just as people vary in height, pain tolerance, or susceptibility to sunburn, so, too, people vary in their emotional sensitivity to their environment.

- When your emotional boundaries are "thin," you will tend to react readily to the environment in which you find yourself. In a way you *fuse* with it, becoming like it. That leads to your being suggestible as you're unduly influenced by what is going on around you.

- If you are a person whose feelings are more developed than your thinking, you will tend to be influenced in situations where you *know* better.

What not to do:

Do not allow yourself to get in trouble because of your suggestibility.

What to do:

1. Recognize how you are naturally constructed, and do what you need to do to be in charge of your feelings and actions.

2. Accept the fact, in a nonjudgmental way, that you have a high level of sensitivity with less ability to self-protect emotionally than a lot of people. Acknowledge that you find it hard to "screen out" the emotional tone that surrounds you.

3. Tell yourself that you are neither good nor bad because of the way your emotional boundaries are easily penetrated.

4. Realize you can heighten your awareness about this and learn to get in charge of it.

5. When you enter a group, make a note about how you feel and what the tone of the group is. You may notice, for example, that there is a lot of frenzied energy. Or maybe individuals in the group are angry. Not all group energy is negative. You may move into an environment that feels peaceful and calm, and it will help you become peaceful and calm.

6. Consciously decide whether you want to let yourself pick up the energy of the group.

7. If you don't, visualize a barrier around you that keeps you emotionally separate. Or you may want to imagine you are somewhere else that has the feeling tone you desire. Meditation will help you deal with the group. Stay alert and pay attention to your breathing.

View from the Cliff

8. Know that your heightened awareness can protect you, making up for your thin boundaries.

What makes this hard to do:

Not everyone is susceptible to the effects of their environment. As a result, others may not be able to empathize with you. They may even scold you or put you down because of your suggestibility. You will certainly be held responsible for it.

TAKING THINGS PERSONALLY

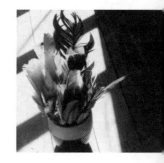

DO YOU TEND TO TAKE THINGS PERSONALLY?

The checkout person at the store glowers at you when you ask a question about the specials for this week—as if you should have known. Her look crucifies you, and you feel bad the rest of the day.

Why this happens:

- Because of your inborn sensitivity, you feel everything keenly. That makes you extremely empathic—a trait that yields compassion, caring,

and openness to others. It also means you get your feelings hurt easily.

- Being someone who tends to look at the whole scene rather than the individual aspects of what's going on, you don't differentiate between what you are and are not responsible for. So when something goes wrong, you take it personally.

- Because of your type of brain construction, you tend also to *become one* with everyone you meet. You become immersed in the person's attitude and demeanor. This means you take personally how others respond to you.

■ Perhaps you haven't yet learned that it's okay to be naïve, or ignorant, or that there's nothing wrong with making a mistake.

■ Your sensitive nature also makes you vulnerable to hurt from being scolded, chastised, shamed, judged, and emotionally attacked.

■ You may not have learned to see another person as insensitive and boorish. Others have problems and feelings of their own that they are not taking responsibility for and, therefore, are unintentionally dumping on anyone who happens to be around.

What not to do:

Do not take everything personally that happens to and around you.

What to do:

1. Adjust for your natural style of brain construction so you are protected from the hurt of taking everything personally.

2. Look honestly at yourself to determine how identified you become in what others say and do. Ask, "What's happening here?"

3. When another person jumps on you, think through the situation so you can realize that the person may be stressed or feeling out of control. After all, that's why people are anxious, depressed, and angry even when they don't express it clearly. It's also why someone jumps on another person. It probably has little to do with you.

4. Don't bother to tell yourself not to

Using and Protecting Your Sensitivity

take things personally. That's like telling your skin to not sunburn if you're fair-complected.

5. Engage your thinking and separate out your feelings for a moment. Ask yourself, "What more could I have done to make the outcome better?"

6. Know you have choices. You can stop any transaction or situation that is uncomfortable and walk out. You can ignore a look or simply ask the person, "Are you having a bad day?" Only turn the tables if you feel strong enough to deal with this obviously stressed person. If you don't, select the first choice, knowing that you can always become supportive of others when you feel stronger within yourself. Take care of yourself first.

7. Either journal about your feelings or talk them out with a friend if you are feeling bad. Then let them go. If there is something you can change, do so the next time around.

Otherwise, chalk up what happened to experience.

8. Later, if you would like to work more with your reaction, you can continue doing the following. Get a mental picture of yourself as a young child. No, you're not acting childish now. But there is a likelihood that in addition to being thin-skinned, you also reacted so strongly because you've had some previous experiences that have left emotional memories from previous *wounds*. The Wounded You recognized a previously hurtful situation. It's a memory thing. You bumped into an old emotional bruise.

9. Self-nurture that part. Let yourself know you will protect that part. Talk to the wonderful part of you saying, "I'm sorry you were hurt. There, there, it'll be okay." Then add, "I'll take care of you now," as if you're talking to a young child. Continue saying, "We can get out of here now. Come on."

10. If you want to take one more step, you can look in your mind's eye at the person or persons who created the bruise in the first place. Ask yourself what that person needed. After all, people are hurtful because they need something and don't know another way to get it. It could be anything from his or her fear of failure to a need to control everything, which is also a reaction to the fear of being helpless and out of control.

11. Consider forgiving that person for not doing better originally. You can do this if you know that you won't let your vulnerable part be hurt again. You are now in charge.

What makes this hard to do:

You aren't likely to be able to completely change taking things personally. But by becoming aware of how you are made, you can spare yourself continued hurt and pain.

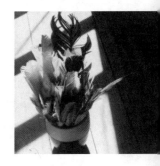

DEFENDING THE UNDERDOG

DO YOU FREQUENTLY FIND YOURSELF DEFENDING THE UNDERDOG?

You assert yourself, sometimes quite loudly, on behalf of people who have less than you. You rescue stray animals and cry over dead butterflies. You've even been known to get in a fight to defend someone who is being taken advantage of. Though you could stay out of trouble by minding your own business, you simply can't stand it when someone uses their authority unfairly or treats people poorly. You probably could make more money, working in a job that doesn't deal with society's underdogs. You may have even lost a job or compromised a relationship because of how you feel and believe.

Why this happens:

- Your innate sensitivity means you are very, very empathic. You hurt when other people hurt.

- It's possible that your own memories of having been hurt are stimulated when you're around a situation where someone or something is hurt or wronged. The Wounded You is touched.

- As a big picture person, you are likely to see others, even animals, as an important part of your life—kind of one big family.

- Sometimes you hurt so much that you have to do something to remedy the situation. After all, as a kinesthenic person, you will tend to "take action" when a cause demands it.

- Finally, your strong feelings mean you lead with your heart, not your head.

What not to do:

Do not stop feeling or become dulled to the hurtful things in the world. Do not, however, let yourself drown in another person's problems.

What to do:

1. Even though you feel first, do not automatically act upon those feelings. Let a little time pass before you act.

2. Become aware of what you're feeling and why. Realize you are likely to take on the feelings of another person because you are very empathic. (See Catching Another's Feelings, p. 171.)

3. Find ways to use your feelings to identify a situation that is wrong.

4. Then analyze those feelings and begin to think about what might be the most efficient way to act. In the long run, you can run around using up a lot of time without making much headway if you don't think first. And that behavior all too easily leads to burnout. Then no one gains.

5. It can be very noble, even heroic, to put your own well-being on the line for another person. But before you do, be sure that is the best move to make for both of you. After all, if you both drown, there's no one left to tell the tale. Think about the

Using and Protecting Your Sensitivity

implication of what you do. Then do the most you can for the other person while considering how much you want to jeopardize your own position.

You must be careful that you don't do anything for another person that the person can do for himself or herself. If you do, you enable that person to stay inadequate and dependent. And, ultimately, you're taking advantage of the person so you can look good or not deal with your own emotional issues.

It's up to you how much you choose to sacrifice. Just be sure you've thought through your decision. This reflects the marriage of your heart and mind.

6. Try taking a crisis intervention course. Through it you can learn how to help others effectively.

7. Consider multiple options to help others. You can become involved personally by becoming a teacher, mentor, or protector. You can speak out for a cause. You can create an organization or plan a remedy for a situation. You can write about the problem or become a fundraiser not only for the person or situation but for others facing the same issue.

8. You must also learn to protect your sensitive feelings so you don't "burn out." For example, if you rescue animals, you may begin with one or two, but pretty soon have ten or twelve. You may volunteer at the animal shelter once a week, then twice a week. Next you may begin to worry about all the poor animals on days when you're not there. Finally you decide to quit your job and work with the animals five days a week and eventually start going in on weekends, too.

When you're dealing with a perennial problem, you have to realize you can't save the world. And you must set limits on the part you will do so you don't burn out, becoming totally ineffective.

9. Limit your exposure to problems. This may mean limiting the amount of television you watch and the news stories you read.

What makes this hard to do:

It's very hard for sensitive, kinesthenic people to ignore hurt and injustice. It's hard to face the fact that each of us has limitations with regard to how much we can accomplish in a lifetime to make things right. Know what you can reasonably do. Do it. Then let go of the rest.

FEELING OVERWHELMED

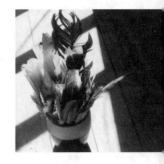

DO YOU FEEL OVERWHELMED, NEARING PANIC IN NEW AND CROWDED SITUATIONS?

You are entering a room full of people you've never met. The task is to mix and mingle. You feel overwhelmed, confused, and want to get out of there.

Why this happens:

- A common reason this happens is because of something called "flooding." Because you see the big picture first before noticing details, you can become easily overwhelmed with

stimulation in new situations.

- When The True You is extremely sensitive, you tend to deeply experience what you see, feel, hear, and sense, both physically and intuitively. When there is so much coming too fast for you to be able to process through it right away, you become flooded with stimulation. It takes time to see the patterns created by the new situation and to figure out how things are working.

- When you have a job to do, this

focuses your attention and you are better able to orient yourself. When you have directions or plans that guide you, you do better. But caught off guard or being unclear about your role or direction, you encounter an unpleasant experience.

What not to do:

Do not press yourself to overcome your discomfort by forcing yourself prematurely into a new situation. Do not automatically think there is something pathologically wrong with you that requires medication and extensive therapy.

What to do:

1. Create an approach that fits you when encountering new and stimulating situations.

2. Back up against the nearest wall, lean against it for support, and simply wait. Give yourself time to see what's going on. Either you'll see someone you want to talk to, or something you want to do, or someone will come over to talk to you. That's the beginning. You're on your way.

3. Have a job to do, something you planned out ahead of time. If you are quite edgy about these situations, the job needs to involve something more tangible than making conversation with others. For example, you may pass out brochures or appetizers, check people in, or help in the serving line.

What makes this hard to do:

When you believe that *everyone* automatically knows what to do when they enter a room, you'll assume there is something wrong with you because you don't. You will have to unlearn your old perception of yourself. That can take time, but you can do it.

TAKING THE CHAOS OUT OF MEETINGS

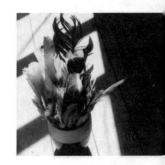

DO YOU HAVE A HARD TIME KNOWING WHAT IS GOING ON DURING MEETINGS OR GATHERINGS?

You join an organization because you are interested in what they do, but when you attend the first meeting, you feel lost. You don't know what to do to get started. You wonder how others seem to know what to do even though they are new, too.

Why this happens:

■ Because you have to figure out the patterns and processes involved, in the gathering it will take you time to sort through the agendas at hand.

■ You see the big picture, and that means there's a lot to look at all at once. Remember that many people who start something new don't see as broadly as you do. That is neither good nor bad. It just is.

■ Besides having to figure out about the activity that brought you to the meeting, you are going to be inundated with everyone's feelings and personal agendas. This is because you are innately sensitive to everything around you.

What not to do:

Do not avoid groups.

What to do:

1. Take your time adjusting to a new group. Study the people who are there. What roles do they seem to be playing? Look for group needs that are unfulfilled. Then notice where your skills might be needed.

2. Think about why you're there and what *you* want to accomplish.

3. Notice who has the power in the group.

4. Pay attention to individuals to whom you are drawn.

5. Ask questions that come to your mind, drawing others out so you can find how the group works.

6. Be willing to take on a small helper's job initially so you can gain more time to figure out all the various aspects of the group.

7. Know your talents are important. The group will need your skills, whatever they are. When you're ready, make your contributions.

8. If all else fails, start your own group and let everyone else fit into it.

What makes this hard to do:

Impatience and feelings that you should know what is happening will make it hard for you to enter a new group situation. You will eventually become an asset to the group as you see patterns in the initial chaos.

TRAVELING WITHOUT STRESS

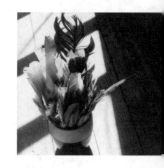

DOES IT TAKE YOU A WHILE ON VACATIONS TO FIGURE OUT HOW TO RELAX AND HAVE FUN?

Does traveling seem like work at times, causing you stress even though you like adventure and scouting out new places? It's just that it takes you time to learn the ropes, and you may feel confused and uncomfortable when you're in airports, bus and train stations, and any other setting where there are a lot of people milling around.

You've tried preplanned tours, but you always seem to want to do some-thing different from the crowd. So you need to come up with ways to have fun without too much work.

Why this happens:

■ Traveling means you must change from your regular routine. Changes take time and effort for everyone, but sensitive people feel the changes particularly keenly.

■ Though you can get into the groove of traveling (moving and changing), you must find your own rhythm first and that takes time.

- Once you've "gotten in the groove," you can turn your attention to having fun.

- Preplanned tours may not work well for you because your adventurous self will want to guide you to your own types of pleasure. You must listen to your feelings for this to work. And that means you have to pay attention to your feelings first.

What not to do:

Do not put yourself in a situation that controls you so you lose touch with your natural rhythm.

What to do:

1. Do take your time and find your own rhythm in whatever kind of vacation you choose to undertake.

2. In one kind of trip you spontaneously take off and simply follow your nose. Perhaps you flip a coin. If it lands on heads, you turn left (in your car, motorcycle, or bike). If it lands on tails, you turn right. You go when you want to and stop when you want to. If this sounds fun, even interesting, do it.

3. Prepare for a number of eventualities. Pack enough food in your vehicle to last a few days. Have several changes of clothes. Take some "camping gear" or enough money to rent a place from time to time. Take good maps or get them along the way.

4. Know ahead of time how long you can/will be gone. Simply turn around when you've used up half of your time.

5. Ask "locals" where the good places are to eat and the interesting activities are happening.

6. Talk to people along the way.

7. Take a journal, paints, camera, or

whatever creative materials you like.

8. Stay flexible, always willing to change your plans.

9. In the second form of traveling, you follow a preplanned agenda of your own making. Here you have some reservations with deadlines for arrival and departure. You may want to have a friend who is more linear than you help you lay out the itinerary ahead of time. Also consider a traveling companion who has planning skills you don't have.

   Then when you get to a new place, let that friend take over for a while until you start to feel comfortable. If you are alone, give yourself time to wander around and get the lay of the land.

10. Plan a couple of extra days for "getting adjusted time."

11. Do not push yourself initially.

12. Do not spend a lot of money right away until you know the options that are available.

13. Do not necessarily follow the regimen that most tourists who go to the area follow. You are likely to want to create a trip that spends more time in one place than most people do and then skip other "typical" tourist sites.

14. Talk to more than one person about your options.

15. You may want to hire a guide initially to get the overview so you know what your options are after you've gotten the big picture.

16. When you are in a crowded place, be willing to ask questions—lots of questions.

17. Remember to breathe calmly and deeply, shut your eyes, and remember who you are and that you are

simply a traveler at this time who is having an adventure. Stay in the present rather than worrying about what you'll do next and next and next.

18. Oh yes, and remember that the point is to have a good time. And only you can determine how you will fulfill that agenda by doing what you want.

19. If you're traveling with someone with whom you're not compatible, you will probably be frustrated. Consider splitting up for a while so you can each do what you like.

20. If you like structure and aren't interested in creating it yourself, consider a cruise with lots of things to do but that has a definite framework to support you.

What makes this hard to do:

If you try to do too much in one trip, you'll overload yourself. If you turn your power over to someone else and begin to do things you don't want to do, you will begin to feel bad. Take your power back.

If you believe that trips and vacations are always wonderful and never fraught with problems, you are likely to be disappointed. Take interest in all that happens at the time it's happening instead of overfocusing on the goal.

Using and Protecting Your Sensitivity

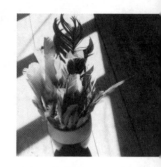

INTERRUPTING CONVERSATIONS

DO YOU FIND YOURSELF "GETTING INTO TROUBLE" BECAUSE YOU DON'T MIND YOUR OWN BUSINESS?

You overhear two people talking. One asks the other a question for which you have an answer. Unasked, you interrupt them with the answer. As a result, you are told to "mind your own business."

Why this happens:

- Common reasons you do not exercise the boundaries and limits others seem to see are because you focus more on the content of what is happening than the details. You probably focus more on the question than a detail like whom the question was addressed to. A person with a more linear style of brain construction is likely to see the situation in the opposite way.

- You may also have feelings of inadequacy and be trying to prove to others and yourself that you are knowledgeable.

What not to do:

Don't interrupt and take responsibility for what hasn't been asked of you.

What to do:

1. Learn to recognize other people's business and ask yourself if you want to cross into their turf.

2. Heighten your awareness. Right now commit to paying attention to how you act around other people.

3. Ask yourself whether you cut people off or intrude in their business.

4. Be honest with yourself. It may take time, but you'll get the knack of doing this.

5. Focus on the people around you.

6. Ask yourself, "Who asked the question? Did that person address the question to me?"

7. Wait. Count to ten, if you must, before you say anything.

8. Observe whether the person asked is quiet because he or she is thinking. Realize that people problem-solve at different rates. You may be able to come up with answers at lightning speed. But if another person can't, don't jump in prematurely.

9. If the person doesn't know the answer, you may then, and only then, ask if input from you would be welcomed. You need permission to join the conversation if you are not already a part of it.

10. Don't push the situation if the people involved ignore you or change the subject. Remember, this wasn't your situation in the beginning and you can only join in if you are invited.

11. If you have feelings of inadequacy, check to see if you are trying to

impress someone with what you know or are trying to prove to yourself that you're smart.

12. Sense whether you are feeling uneasy in your stomach or lightheaded. Note how your emotions feel. Are you afraid that you'll never amount to anything? Do you feel depressed because you feel you're not as smart as other people?

13. Realize that you learned these thoughts and feelings in error. The thoughts are untrue. You are not inadequate.

14. Visualize yourself when you were younger and talk to yourself as a good parent would reassure a small child. Be a good self-parent to yourself.

15. Tell yourself that you are a winner, as valuable and smart as anyone else.

16. Say "thank you" to yourself for being good to yourself.

What makes this hard to do:

Habits are hard to break. But remember, this is your first day committed to changing the habit of stepping into other people's territory. You can do it. Just take one step at a time. It doesn't matter if you don't do it overnight.

BORROWING WITHOUT PERMISSION

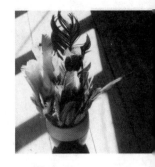

DO YOU SOMETIMES GET INTO TROUBLE BORROWING THINGS WITHOUT PERMISSION?

You are happy to share what you have at home and on the job. But when you *borrow* a coworker's tools without first asking, he gets angry with you. The same thing happened when you wore your brother's shirt without asking. You don't understand it. You take care of things and are very responsible about returning them.

Why this happens:

■ With your eye on the goal, you forget the steps needed to reach it. Attention to the big picture does you in as you fail to see or acknowledge the details—details others consider important. In this case, the goal is getting something done at work or dressing well for an occasion. The steps include who "owns" the article needed to reach the goal.

■ Because you're a kinesthenic person, one whose action skills are highly developed, you may forget that when an action intrudes on another's turf, it crosses that person's physical boundaries.

- Tools, clothes, and all kinds of items belong to their owner, not you. In a culture that has strong guidelines for ownership, crossing these boundaries is considered impolite and wrong.

- If you feel emotionally close to another person, you may assume that what belongs to that person is automatically available to you and the person won't mind. You probably wouldn't mind if the tables were turned, so you can't imagine their minding. Thinking this way means you experience things globally. By definition, seeing things globally automatically means you see them without limits and boundaries. So you may simply not see limits that others see.

What not to do:

Do not continue to ignore physical boundaries, taking what doesn't officially belong to you. But do not brand yourself as a bad person either.

What to do:

1. Learn how to control the global tendencies that are so much a part of you so you can use them when and where they are appropriate and restrain them when necessary.

2. Immediately realize that you can get in big trouble socially and even legally if you take what doesn't belong to you. Other people may disapprove of this behavior and feel they need to do something about it.

3. When you want something, stop and think what individual steps are needed for you to get what you want.

4. Practice looking around your workspace and through your personal belongings to note what belongs to

you. Notice what belongs to others. This will begin to create two categories in your mind: "Mine" and "others."

5. Either return anything that is not yours or reaffirm your use of it with the person.

6. Make a habit of respectfully asking to use things that belong to someone else, even if that person is a family member or close friend who you're sure won't mind. It's just good practice.

What makes this hard to do:

Probably lack of awareness is the biggest obstacle you face in implementing a willingness to respect what belongs to others. Fortunately this is something you can work on.

RESPECTING JOB BOUNDARIES

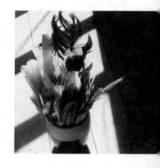

DO YOU IRRITATE PEOPLE AT WORK BY MIXING INTO THEIR BUSINESS?

Even though your job assignment is clear-cut, you find you frequently want to give input to coworkers or use an idea they're working on. You may be so focused on getting your job done that you don't respect others' territorial rights at work. Some people love your approach. Others get offended and may even go so far as to tell you to mind your own business.

Why this happens:

- In reality, you are likely to be very responsible. But if you focus on the goal of accomplishing the job that is given you rather than on *how* it is to be done, or who has the power with respect to various aspects of the project, you are likely to step on someone's toes, alienating coworkers.

- You may forget when you don't have responsibility for a project that you have no inherent right to make decisions that affect another person. Neither do you have the right to use something they have been working on unless they offer it to you.

- Anyone who pays more attention to details than the process of getting something done will likely get upset when you overlook the boundaries between what they're responsible for and what you are responsible for.

What not to do:

Do not overlook others' territorial rights. Remember that not everyone is constructed the way you are. Some are very serious and territorial about their work areas, ideas, and skills.

What to do:

1. Know the limits of your job and the tolerance of your coworkers for crossing those limits.

2. Know clearly what assignment or job you're fulfilling and who's in charge. That will give you information about who has the power in any situation.

3. Observe how flexible individuals are. Notice whether the organization reinforces shared work versus expecting each person to do his or her own task.

4. Discover how territorial your coworkers are. Ask yourself how much they guard what they are responsible for. This could be anything from materials to space to ideas.

5. Ask before borrowing things, assignments, or time from a coworker. Also ask about giving to another department or person.

6. Be sensitive to others' responses to your offers to lend ideas, equipment, or time. Not everyone sees your generosity as valuable. Don't push yourself on someone. Read their lack of response as an indicator that they are probably not interested in your offer but don't know how to say no.

7. Give anyone from whom you borrow acknowledgment for the role he or she plays in the final creation or project.

8. Say, "Thank you."

9. If you are extremely creative and carry the big vision of whatever you do, you might want to consider self-employment, where you are the one in charge. That way you can put things together in unique combinations. You're free to do this as much as you like with your own business.

Or you may choose to look for a creative partnership or group that is clearly open to working in a boundary-hopping style.

What makes this hard to do:

You may get focused exclusively on the process of reaching your goal, caught up as you are in the creative process. Or you may feel angry that other people "get in the way" of what you consider most important.

HUGGING AND TOUCHING OTHERS

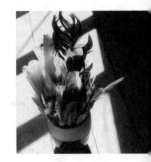

DO OTHER PEOPLE SOMETIMES PULL AWAY BECAUSE YOU ARE MORE PHYSICALLY EXPRESSIVE THAN THEY ARE?

You want to be friendly, so you hug someone who, to your surprise, stiffens or pulls away from you. You don't mean any harm. But you don't understand the reaction.

You have noticed how sensitive you are to certain kinds of touch. You wonder if it's the same thing.

Why this happens:

■ As an expressive, kinesthenic person whose exuberant feelings abound, you may forget or even be unaware that not everyone is comfortable with the way you naturally express yourself.

■ You may feel that another person's hesitation means they don't like you. But that is not necessarily true. Taking other people's responses personally is due to the way you see the world. (See Taking Things Personally, p. 178.)

■ Not everyone likes the same kind of

touch. Being extremely physically sensitive, you and others may have distinct preferences for how you are touched and what touches your skin. Brain construction dictates these levels of sensitivity.

- You may be accused of being insensitive to others' feelings when, in reality, you may have only learned to ignore feeling altogether.

  Often very sensitive babies and children are innocently hurt—even the roughness of fabric or the tags on clothes hurt. Those experiences can teach a child to disregard his own and others' physical nature.

- Not everyone shows friendliness physically.

What not to do:

Do not ignore another's reactions to you.

What to do:

1. Learn how to express your friendliness while taking another person's preferences into account.

2. Right now, think about the people you know. Rank them according to how much you think they like being hugged or touched. This may range from "Not at all" to "Lots."

3. Check with a few of the people with whom you have a close relationship. This will help you develop sensitivity to other people's preferences.

4. When you like someone, begin to ask yourself whether you think that person would like to be hugged or touched.

5. Begin to read body language. Notice:

   Does the person pull away from you or lean toward you when you're talking?

Does the person talk only about *things* or does he or she also talk about feelings and how he or she feels?

Does the person seem like an emotionally warm person or a cool one?

Does the person make eye contact with you?

6. If you're unsure whether a person will like being touched or hugged, ask, "Do you like hugs?" Notice whether the person reaches toward you enthusiastically or pulls back or looks restrained. Respect the answer.

7. If you are keenly sensitive to another's energy, simply stop and ask yourself how you sense the person. Then trust what you sense.

8. Become aware of your own sensitivity to touch and clearly distinguish what you like and dislike.

9. Begin practicing sharing your preferences with others. You will feel better as a result and you will help others learn to express their preferences.

What makes this hard to do:

It's hard to realize that not everyone likes what you do. And it may also mean you won't always be able to get what you like. That's hard to give up.

It's also difficult to read another person if you expect the person to be a certain way and then he or she is not. An example of this would be a long-lost relative or an in-law whom you don't know well. You consider both *family*. But remember, just because they're family doesn't mean they like what you like or think the way you think.

GETTING COMFORTABLE WITH TOUCH

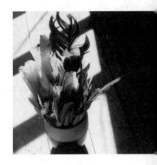

DO YOU FIND IT HARD TO LET YOUR PARTNER KNOW WHAT PLEASES YOU SEXUALLY?

You love your significant other deeply. You are glad you're with your partner. But you're struggling a little sexually. You are attracted to him or her and like sex, but there are little things that bother you—well, actually, things they do that drive you up the wall.

He likes to stroke your skin, but after a few sweeps of his hand, you've had enough. You can tell he's trying hard to please you when he engages in a lot of foreplay, but it gets on your nerves. And the pressure of his body on yours often feels too heavy. Even having him put his arm around your shoulder may make you feel weighted down, so much so that you want him to remove it.

You feel badly about how you feel. You feel foolish that you react the way you do. And worst of all, you don't know how to talk to him about all of this without hurting his feelings. You'd never want to do that.

Why this happens:

■ Each of us has different sensitivity to the amount and type of touch we prefer.

■ The way in which the sensation of touch feels has nothing to do with how much we love a partner.

■ You cannot tell by looking at someone what kind of touching and how much the person likes and wants.

■ There is generally a myth in this culture that makes couples think they ought to automatically know what each other likes and wants if they *love* one another.

■ Words must convey the message. And in the beginning of an intimate relationship you must talk, otherwise the displeasure will build into a giant block to intimacy if your feelings and preferences go unspoken.

■ There is no right or wrong way of approaching lovemaking as long as both people desire the means.

What not to do:

Do not fail to communicate likes and dislikes about intimate touch.

What to do:

1. Learn to communicate your preferences to your partner, clearly and without judgment.

2. Begin by telling the other person how much you love them and that you are excited about exploring how you can bring one another pleasure.

3. Let inquisitiveness and curiosity be your guiding map. Don't assume you ought to know what to do or that there is *one* way of doing it.

4. If you know you are sensitive to touch, tell your partner right away. Have this conversation when you are

Using and Protecting Your Sensitivity

on sexually neutral ground, not when either of you is aroused.

You might say something like, "I've always been very sensitive to touch, honey, kind of like the princess in the *Princess and the Pea* fairy tale in which a woman was known to be a true princess if she could feel a pea underneath thirteen mattresses." Then, you may feel like smiling and adding, "So I guess I'm your princess."

Continue saying, "I like to be touched in some ways, and I can't stand to be touched in others. This has nothing to do with you. I promise. It's how I'm made."

Then proceed to share what you know about yourself, what you like and dislike. Show him. For example, maybe you like to be held firmly, but hate to be tapped. Let him know if you like a little stroking but not a lot. Perhaps you say, "I really like it when you. . . ."

5. If your partner has already unwittingly transgressed your pleasure zone, doing something you don't like, tell them so, adding that they had no way of knowing. Reflect back their intention, saying, "I love that you want to please me." Then ask them to do something else to show the same affection. For example, if he or she has a habit of putting their arm around your shoulders, say, "I want you to hug me. Will you put your arms around my waist? I'd like that."

6. More than likely, your lover will have a questioning look on his face. When you see it, ask, "Would you like to know why?" He'll probably say yes, and you can tell him. "My shoulders are very sensitive to pressure and it feels as if there is a lot of weight pressing me down. I know your intent is to do something nice for me, so we need to find a way to do that that works for me."

7. Make "I" statements, that is, take

responsibility for how you feel instead of making "you" statements. "You press down too hard" puts the responsibility for the problem on your partner. That's very different from saying, "I don't feel good with pressure on my shoulders."

8. Tell him "thank you" for being understanding. Then enjoy your mutually satisfying intimacy. You may have to guide him and his love-making from time to time, just as he will need to guide you. That's a natural part of bringing pleasure to one another. Rejoice as you continue to explore and find what works and what doesn't. Have fun!

9. If your honey gets hurt feelings, just say, "This is my deal. It's only the way in which my brain and nerves are constructed. It's no reflection on you."

10. If he's critical of you or says you *shouldn't* be so sensitive, say, "I'm as sensitive as I am. It's a part of me. I hope you can understand and respect my wishes."

11. If he criticizes or shames you further, strongly consider getting out of the relationship quickly. Your desires and rights must be appreciated and honored. Besides, he's not available for a mutually pleasuring relation-ship.

What makes this hard to do:

Most often it's the fear that you're not doing sex *right* that gets in the way, as you have an unrealistic expectation that true lovers and experienced sexual partners will automatically know what to do. There's also the fear that the other person won't continue to love you if you say anything. Actually, healthy true love can only grow with communication and sharing.

Using and Protecting Your Sensitivity

FEELING IN THE MOOD FOR SEX

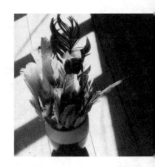

DO YOU WONDER WHY YOU HAVE TO "FEEL IN THE MOOD" FOR LOVEMAKING, WHILE SOME PEOPLE SEEM TO BE ABLE TO ENJOY SEX REGARDLESS OF WHAT THEIR DAY HAS BEEN LIKE?

You've noticed how your wife is almost always ready for lovemaking, but you're not. It's not that you don't like sex. You do, passionately—at times. It's not that you don't love your wife and like to have sex with her. You adore her and cherish intimate time spent with her.

But if you've had a stressful day, gotten your feelings hurt at work, or are worried, you just aren't in the mood for sex. Though your wife also has a stressful job, even more than you, she seems to go through the day without it getting her down nearly so much as your job gets you down. She simply lets it roll off her back. She doesn't take things that happen personally. She has feelings, but they don't seem to rule her life and moods as yours do, and they certainly don't affect her sexual appetite.

You wonder if there is something wrong with you.

Why this happens:

- Feelings-oriented people feel first rather than think about what is happening to them. If you're this way, you wear your feelings on your sleeve and are particularly susceptible to the effects of stress, hurt, and worry. You can't just *put your feeling aside.*

- Being sensitive to feelings means you will not be able to easily, if at all, override your feelings, especially when you're engaging in something like sex that also involves your feelings. Genuine intimate communication is heart-based. It touches your feelings deeply. So you must be "in the mood," if you're a feelings-oriented person.

What not to do:

Do not override your feelings because you think you *should.* Of course, don't wallow in them either.

What to do:

1. Sensitively assess your needs and those of your mate, using your good thinking mind to decide whether to proceed at a given time or delay lovemaking between you.

2. Assess yourself during a neutral time when you're not making love. Ask yourself, "How sensitive am I to feelings and what happens to me when I'm stressed?" Do you take to heart what other people say or do? Does your mood shift, based on what's going on around you? Be sure to not judge your answers to these questions.

3. Also, in a neutral time, talk with your spouse. Share what you've discovered about yourself. Then ask your spouse to consider the same questions with regard to himself or herself. find out how your spouse is affected by stress and what gets him or her down. Discuss the similarities and differences without criticism or judgment.

4. Devise a set of mental yardsticks to reflect what each of you desires. For example, you might use a scale numbered one to ten to measure the desire each of you has for sex. A one means "I don't want to have sex at all." Ten means "I'm dying to have sex." Let's suppose you rate yourself at a three and your spouse rates himself or herself at a seven. With these scores, you have a tangible guide to help you both decide what to do at this moment.

5. Clearly, without apology, compare your scale results with your partner's.

6. When your partner is fairly eager for sexual relations and you are lukewarm, you need to decide whether you may be able to diffuse your stress after some time or activities. For example, you might do some physical exercise, talk or journal through your feelings, meditate, have your partner give you a back rub, listen to music, read the newspaper, or whatever. Perhaps you'll be able to drain off the stressful feelings. Then you'll feel ready and eager to shift your attention to enjoying relations with your partner.

7. If you can't or don't want to get beyond your feelings at this time, say so. "I am not going to be able to get past my feelings right now." You might also say, "This is not a good time for me to enjoy sex with you. I'm sorry."

8. Then, in the spirit of helping your partner get his or her needs met even though you don't want to have sex right then, ask what you can do for your partner. Make suggestions that you are willing to do. You might suggest getting together at a later time. Or if he or she is feeling very sexually aroused, volunteer to engage for his or her enjoyment. It can be extremely satisfying to bring your partner pleasure without your being sexually aroused. Your pleasure comes from bringing him or her pleasure.

9. If you absolutely do not want to engage in any stimulating involvement, say so and perhaps simply hold your partner tenderly. The lack of resolution can be a tender occurrence between you. Though lovers want to be there for each other, it simply is not always possible. Acknowledging the limits of your humanness can create a profound sharing, if it's done between two emotionally healthy individuals who understand their own and another's limitations. It can be a sweet time.

10. Under no circumstances make the result of your feelings your spouse's problem, such as by saying, "Why do *you* always want sex? *You* know I'm tired after work!" This puts the *blame* or responsibility onto him or her.

11. By the same token, do not let your spouse blame you for the way you are feeling and choosing to act as a result. Sexual relations are a mutually consenting enterprise, freely entered into by both partners. No blackmail, accusations, demands, or forced activities. Shaming and blaming are not a part of a loving relationship. They are signs that an individual needs help with learning acceptable ways to get his or her needs met without hurting another person.

What makes this hard to do:

Many people come into intimate relationships without having learned how to communicate and resolve differences. There is also a lot of "illusion" and fantasy surrounding sex in our culture. It is not usually seen as a natural, mutually enjoyable, freedom-of-choice activity.

Fear plays a big role in individuals not caringly and gently speaking honestly about their needs. Fear of being left or disapproved of and feeling guilty are the most common reasons for people not communicating their needs. A healthy, loving relationship is never based on fear. Don't use it. Don't accept it.

Using and Protecting Your Sensitivity

FACING DENTISTS AND SHOTS

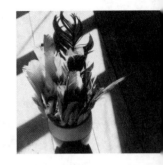

DO YOU ABHOR THE THOUGHT OF GOING TO A DENTIST OR GETTING A SHOT?

Your periodic dental exam is coming up and, immediately, you think of a dozen reasons to put it off. You're an adult, generally courageous and willing and able to face danger and threats head-on. But not when it comes to facing "the drill," "the shot," or even "the needle prick."

It's not just going to the dentist, though, that causes you trouble. Last week you had to go to the doctor to give a blood sample and you nearly passed out. If you had looked at the needle, you'd have been a "goner."

As if your feelings aren't bad enough, you've been scolded and shamed about your reactions. You've heard, "You're acting like a baby," and "Don't be so sensitive." You want to scream, "Well, maybe I am a baby. So what!" You haven't managed to outgrow your fears, and you sure haven't been able to put mind over matter.

Why this happens:

- Bodily sensitivity is determined by

factors in your brain that are out of your control.

- Degrees of sensitivity vary greatly from one person to another. Pain generally is considered a subjective experience. However, people who are particularly sensitive to all stimuli may actually feel more pain than those who are less sensitive. You may be one of those people. If you are bothered by the tags in your clothing, imagine your reaction to shots and other bodily intrusions.

- Pain sensitivity doesn't change over time, though you can learn some techniques to help you get through the challenges.

- People who scold and blame others for their reactions either do not understand the differences between people or they are overcompensating because of their own discomfort. Overcompensation happens when people don't face their own emotional reactions. Instead they cast their feelings onto someone else, like you. If a person calls you a baby, in reality, he or she probably feels like a baby but is too ashamed to admit it.

What not to do:

Do not accept the shame put on you or become self-critical.

What to do:

1. Do protect your sensitive self and learn pain management techniques to make you more comfortable.

2. Immediately give yourself permission to be exactly as sensitive as you are. This means you are to stop thinking that you are somehow lacking because of your reactions.

3. Give yourself permission to be out front with others about how you are. Be matter-of-fact, saying, "I'm a sensitive person." With professionals, interview the person before commit-

ting yourself to their care. If they brush you off or don't acknowledge the importance of what you are saying, seek out someone else. Frequently, the professional is simply trying to stick to a schedule that doesn't allow the individualized attention you need. Some professionals are trained in techniques to assist with sensitive patients and clients. Others are not. Choose one who is empathic and understands the issues at hand.

4. Do not hesitate to ask for assistance from a professional to reduce or overcome your reaction to a procedure. Hypnosis and desensitization techniques can turn a scary situation around to one that is quite tolerable. Medication may also be beneficial. Use whatever you are drawn to without feeling guilty or ashamed.

5. Consider taking an advocate with you who understands you. Your advocate can assist you in getting

what you want even if you're in the middle of a procedure. Your companion can also help you deal with your fears. Of course, you have to choose someone who knows what he or she is doing and doesn't feel embarrassed around authority or become nervous in such a situation.

6. To family and friends who may have something negative to say about your sensitivity, simply set limits. "I prefer not to talk about it, and I sure don't want any criticism."

7. Learn self-hypnosis. Take a class or meet with a counselor who teaches this technique. It is simple and will do wonders to help you relax. You'll have a skill of value for life as a result.

What makes this hard to do:

Your own hesitation to stand up for yourself may cause you to suffer emotionally as well as physically.

RELIVING PAST PAIN

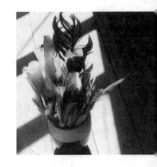

DOES YOUR MIND REPLAY HURTFUL EVENTS OVER AND OVER?

Recently you were criticized and humiliated during a presentation of your work. You had been working on it for a long time and believed in what you were presenting. You were not only told you were wrong, but told you didn't understand the issues. "Get into something else," was a remark that cut you to the core. You had believed keenly in what you were doing, but . . . maybe you were wrong all along. That thought twists your gut and makes you feel hopeless about yourself.

The Wounded You relives pain you experienced long ago when you were told what you did was worthless. You were a kid then and had tried hard but failed. Perhaps you misunderstood an assignment. The kids laughed at you and the teacher scolded you, saying you hadn't been paying attention. You were humiliated. Even today you hear the words clearly in your mind. They resonate through your head ever since your recent humiliation. When you aren't hearing, feeling, and thinking about the pain, you feel confused and numb. You even have been having trouble sleeping.

Why this happens:

- Traumatic experiences leave their mark on our emotions and intrude into our thought processes. As our minds struggle to deal with unacceptable, painful experiences, the whole ordeal may repeat itself in our minds. Parts of it cycle through our heads like a stuck phonograph needle.

  Usually we think of traumatic events as such things as rape and sexual and physical abuse, wartime experiences, or what happens to someone who is the victim of crime, an accident, or severe illness. But everyday scoldings, criticisms, and humiliations have the same effect on sensitive, emotionally thin-skinned people. Even watching or hearing of these kinds of trauma-producing events or seeing them in a movie or on TV can leave scars on those who are empathic.

- Sensitive people are more likely to suffer traumatic reactions because of what is said to them. This is because more feeling gets through their defensive systems to traumatize them than they can handle. Folks who are able to let things roll of their backs or who look at things from an impersonal perspective suffer fewer traumatic reactions than people whose feelings act as their primary processing mode.

- Sometimes old memories of hurtful situations will trigger a reoccurrence of a past trauma. Let's say your boss criticizes you publicly. You may feel and believe she is wrong, but you react, nonetheless, as if you're being crucified. Long ago you may have suffered an incident that you since *forgot* about until the current resurrection by your boss.

- In an active, creative mind, sometimes the fear of something happening simulates the actual happening, resulting in a trauma reaction.

■ You are likely to experience a trauma reaction if you are brainwashed to believe that The True You is unacceptable or less than wonderful. Therefore, minority people as well as those who don't fit the cultural model of excellence are subjected to trauma-producing beliefs. People whose brain construction is not linear experience this kind of assault to their self-esteem and crippling to their sense of adequacy.

What not to do:

Do not run away from the pain in any fashion or try to numb it with alcohol or drugs (prescription or street).

What to do:

1. Take the steps needed to assist your psyche in truly healing from the trauma. Know that many people have experienced such healing.

2. Immediately stop the wounding. You may say to the person committing the assault, "That's enough." You can hold up your hand, palm toward the person speaking, or you can back off. Leave the room if necessary.

3. Take a deep breath and begin to nurture yourself. You may immediately begin to rock, even while you're standing. You may visualize yourself hugging your vulnerable inner self. Maybe start to hum to yourself. Walk outside. Swing. Use whatever physical soothing feels good to you.

4. Call or go see someone you trust who will simply listen to you and offer support. You do not want someone to problem-solve at this stage. You most definitely do not want someone to tell you what you *should* or *could* have done differently.

5. If your personality is the type that tends to fight, you're likely to immediately criticize and verbally attack the person hurting you. You may put the person down. It's a cover-up for how badly hurt you feel. This is a natural response, though one that

may get you in big trouble and eventually come around to hurt you. It also doesn't solve the true problem, healing The Wounded You.

6. Check with yourself to see if you're ready to decide what you want to do about your healing. If you don't feel ready to do anything, don't do anything.

7. When you're ready to talk out the old wounding, consult a friend, minister, or counselor. Journal the old experience and rewrite the old script so it has a different ending, one that is supportive, healing, and empowering.

   Hypnotherapy can do wonders if the traumatic experience cuts deeply.

8. When you're ready—remember, no rush—begin to look at your current situation objectively. Here are some guidelines in the form of questions to ask.

   Was this a repetitive occurrence with this person? Does this person strike out only at you or at all people? If this is an equal opportunity hammering, you at least know you're not being picked on. On the other hand, if you are the main target of the person's abuse, you know clearly it will probably continue to be aimed directly at you, and discussing the situation is not very likely to yield good results.

   Do the outbursts happen frequently or occasionally? Have they only recently started to happen? If it's recent, it's likely that something stressful is impacting the critic. That's no reason for you to continue to be subjected to the abuse, but at least you can better understand it. And it promises a more optimistic outcome from a discussion. But remember, you don't *have* to have a discussion. You're free to break the ties if you want.

9. Check the amount of all-around stress in your life. If you have a num-

ber of other sources of stress, you may wish to be extra protective of yourself. You may want to distance yourself more than if other parts of your life are stable.

10. No job or relationship is worth being abused. You don't deserve it. And you don't need to put up with it. There are always more jobs and more people with whom to create relationships.

11. Remember, you are your own advocate in the long run, even as you ask others to help you.

12. Sometimes people do not mean to hurt us but do nonetheless. People who are not particularly sensitive to feelings can walk over us with cleats and not know they're doing it. If the person isn't striking out because he or she is wounded and needs to strike out to feel better, you have a stronger likelihood of being able to remain in contact with the person and educate him or her about your sensitivity. Then it would be safe to remain in a relationship with the person.

What makes this hard to do:

If you were abused or criticized as a child, you may not realize there is another way. Get counseling. You never deserved the abuse, and you now have a chance to break the cycle. You're worth it!

Using and Protecting Your Sensitivity

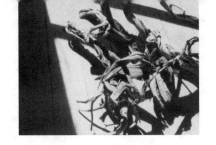

PART FIVE

Succeeding at Work

*As an adult, you can choose
to become your own
authority figure.*

GORDON MACKENZIE

1996

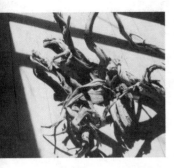

Throughout this book we've been looking at the many ways in which brainstyle impacts the way in which people deal with information and how they feel and behave. We've seen the uniqueness that each of us brings to society. We've watched how our talents and skills are shaped by the processing of our brains. We've learned many ways to utilize our uniqueness in the best interest of our true selves while learning to accommodate to environments that do not readily fit our natural ways, but in which we choose to function in order to achieve outcomes we desire.

The culmination of this understanding and skill building often expresses itself through our work. Whether you're dealing with short-term jobs or long-range career plans, the role played by your particular style of brain construction can give you the edge on success. It can also separate you from achieving your goals.

The True You automatically embraces the unique dreams that make up who you are. To the degree to which you recognize these dreams and follow your desires, you cannot help but succeed if you honor the natural way in which you are constructed. Yet everyday hindrances can act as blocks if you don't see them for what they are and know what to do about them. Ending up disappointed, saddened, and frustrated need not happen when you respect the way in which The True You works.

Through self-understanding and commitment to finding what fits you best on the job, The True You will achieve the focus that will successfully lead you to your goals.

SUFFERING FROM FEELINGS OF INADEQUACY

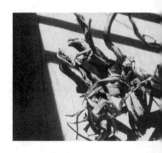

DO YOU SUFFER FROM FEELINGS OF INADEQUACY?

Now that you're married, you thought you'd feel better about yourself. But you still feel inadequate. Your spouse is a successful professional who makes money and keeps track of it. He or she researches and makes all major purchases and the major decisions for the whole family. You feel you don't do anything worthwhile, because you don't earn any money or handle big decisions.

Going back to work doesn't feel like much of an option. When you used to work out of the home, you felt inadequate all of the time. Seems like you worked ten times harder than anyone else just to keep up. Even then you made mistakes and had trouble with deadlines. You never felt caught up— organized. People say how talented you are, creative, and a wonderful person to have on board, but . . . *that* part's easy. *Anyone* can be nice and have ideas. It's your inability to do the *real* work that makes you feel inadequate. You just don't measure up.

Why this happens:

- Different people hold different beliefs. Some people actually believe that one person or set of skills is superior to another. They will justify their beliefs by pointing toward education, amount of money made, social skills, and how serious a person takes life. Yet these are all culturally defined beliefs; they are judgments.

  If someone values "getting ahead" and keeping an orderly home or office, then that person may not realize that not everyone has these same priorities. Another person may value time spent with family and friends or in creative endeavors. Often a person leans in one direction or the other.

- Valuing tasks and skills shaped by a brainstyle different from your own will lead to feelings of inadequacy.

- To the degree you are trying to do work that doesn't naturally fit your brainstyle, no matter what that is, you will need to spend more time accomplishing the same task someone with a good fit to the work spends.

- If you are a hands-on, active, kinesthenic person trying to manage details and keep order, you are not likely to be drawing from your strengths. As a result, you'll be required to work very, very hard just to survive. You'll probably come up short even then. You are likely to feel that you're always catching up and never in control of what you're doing.

- You may also feel inadequate if you are a creative visionary who has trouble translating your visions into reality. It's *so* easy for you to have the vision. It's *so* hard for you to manifest it. This is because you see the completed vision as perfect. But everyday life is not so perfect. Trying to perfectly replicate a dream at home or on the job can cause you to feel frustration and letdown. You still may not achieve a replica of your dream, even with endless hours of trying, though you can achieve a satisfactory replica if you will allow yourself to be realistic and slightly less than perfect.

What not to do:

Do not assume that you have to work so hard all your life or constantly feel inadequate.

What to do:

1. Learn to value the innate gifts you have. The world needs the balance created by all kinds of people working together for the good of all.

2. Figure out why you work so hard and then decide what to do about it.

3. Make two lists. On List 1, note what you like or even love about your jobs at home and in the workplace. Note what is easy for you to do. Note your

strengths. Think of what you accomplish effortlessly on your job. You may not think of these strengths as valuable because they are so easy for you to do.

4. Now figure out on List 2 how much of your time you currently spend doing what you don't like or what feels hard to do.

5. If your natural attributes aren't being readily used, ask why you do what you do. Whose idea is it? Do you want to stay doing these things? How do you want to use your time?

6. Even though you may have spent a lifetime being criticized, consider the possibility that maybe a lot of people hadn't learned to put people first before accomplishments. And they valued one kind of accomplishment higher than another. Think about changing your mind-set.

7. Recognize that there are different

parts of you. There's the frightened part, which is the drudging, over-working part, and there's the part that does things easily. Now, remembering the part of you that does things easily, introduce him or her to the frightened part of you. Tell the frightened part you appreciate how hard he or she has worked for you. Reassure the frightened part that he or she no longer has to attempt to do the things that are too hard. As a result, you don't have to be so frightened.

Then, take a breath and breathe in the new, hopeful attitude and breathe out the old, tense, frightened anger. Continue affirming the positive step with your in-breaths and exhale the old refuse and tension with the out-breaths.

8. Become clear about what you have to offer.

9. If you're a creative visionary with a desire to replicate your dreams in everyday life, you will need to be aware that this is what you're doing. If you let the perfect representation of your desire rule your actions, you can work yourself into a frenzy. If you take the time to think through your situation and what you want to do about it, however, you can get in the driver's seat, making choices that are in your best interest. To do this, consider the audience or recipient of your creative work. Ask,

"How appreciative are they of my finished product?"

"What is the use to which my work is to be put?"

"Do I want or need to put in the amount of time it will take to create near perfect work?"

"Do I have a better use for my time?"

"Are there other projects that are

getting bumped, maybe never to be done, because I'm spending so much time on this one?"

10. Once you've answered these questions, you can make a conscious choice about how you want to spend your time. You can work from your strengths and clearly decide how much time you want to spend manifesting your visions.

11. As a visionary, you must also realize that it takes time for the implementation of your visions to become functional in daily life. Patience is called for.

What makes this hard to do:

Many people think there's status in working exceedingly hard. It's a cultural belief that it is saintly to give 110% all the time. It's not. It's not even possible.

Another attraction to working so hard is that others admire your tenacity without realizing all that work may not be benefiting you or anyone else. You'll need to give up outside approval, face a reevaluation of how you spend your time, and be sure you're living by your own inner beliefs, not those of someone else.

TAKING TESTS

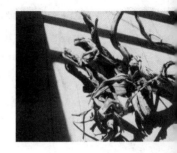

DOES TEST TAKING FEEL NIGHTMARISH TO YOU?

At work recently, you were in line for a promotion, but personnel instigated new procedures that require you to take a test about what you can do and what you know. You've learned it's a multiple-choice test. For as long as you can remember, taking that kind of test has been a nightmare for you. No matter how hard you study or how well you know the information, you do poorly on the test. You'd do better if you were asked to write an essay or show what you can do.

You do your job well. That's why your boss recommended you for promotion, but you fear you won't get the job because of having to take the test.

Why this happens:

- The tests all of us prefer to take, whether at work or school, are those on which we can do well, i.e., they most accurately measure what we know and allow us to show what we know.

- The types of test on which we do

best are a reflection of our style of brain construction.

- To the degree to which you are a person who sees the big picture and recalls the function of something rather its name, you will do poorly on fill-in-the-blank and multiple-choice questions. If you learn and work kinesthenically, you will prefer open-ended, descriptive tests to those requiring you to recall details and labels.

- Answers to multiple-choice tests often have slight variations in content—variations that big picture people have trouble seeing. You are likely to become confused when you're trying to compare details. You know the difference when you're doing your job, but reading about it, out of context, doesn't reflect what you know. If you could write a description of how to do your job, you would probably show clearly the subtleties that you miss on a multiple-choice test.

What not to do:

Do not give up seeking job advancement or an education.

What to do:

1. Learn how to beat the tests or get around them.

2. On the job or in school, you can request that a test of the knowledge needed for your new job be given in a form that shows what you know. Through the Americans with Disabilities Act you have the legal right to be tested in a form that fits your particular style of brain construction. You can ask that the test be given orally or that you demonstrate what you know. (See Returning to College, p. 87, for ADA guidelines and the section on "The Americans with Disabilities Act,"

p. 234, for additional job-related comments.)

3. Often you don't need to go as far as formally instigating ADA. Instead you can ask your current supervisor at work to informally request a dispensation from the formal test. Or the boss or someone who is your supporter may be willing to write a letter of support for you and explain your situation.

4. If you are required to proceed with the testing in its original form, study with someone in the company who is familiar with the test. Go over and over tests like the one you'll be taking. Have your tutor point out the subtle differences between answers so you can learn to think like the person scoring the test.

5. Make a suggestion to those people in the company who are responsible for advancement as well as hiring procedures to become familiar with brain diversity and the assessment needs of various individuals.

6. If you are in training or school, get to know your professor's testing preferences. Even before you register for a class, talk with the person if he or she is accessible. Also ask other students, special needs counselors, and student-friendly professors which professors will fit your learning style best. If at all possible, only take classes from those professors who give tests that your brainstyle allows you to handle successfully.

7. In school, tell your professor about your difficulty taking tests. Ask if you can show her or him in other ways that you can do the work. Ask for extra credit.

What makes this hard to do:

Many people hold an untrue assumption that if you know the material being tested, you will do well on any test.

View from the Cliff

Others simply don't understand that there is a difference between types of tests and not everyone does equally well on all kinds. You must become wise about tests and pass on your wisdom to others.

The Americans with Disabilities Act

1. Everything mentioned in the section entitled "Returning to College" also applies in the workplace. For example, if you are a salesperson and do that job well, you can ask for help with your clerical work. You can ask for flextime so you can come in early or stay late to do your paperwork when the office is quiet.

2. On the job, you generally do not need to make a big deal of *demanding* accommodation. You don't even need to say that you have a special need supported by testing. Simply provide your employer with information about how you can do your job best. Many will accommodate you to that end.

3. Of course, if you feel blocked from doing a good job, your reasonable requests are turned down, or you are poorly rated because of an unaccommodated need, you may wish to use the ADA to get what you need to do a quality job.

ASSESSING JOB HOPPING

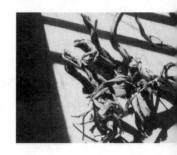

DOES YOUR RESUME HAVE LOTS OF JOBS LISTED, MANY OF WHICH YOU STAYED IN FOR ONLY A SHORT PERIOD?

"Another day, another job" could be your working motto. In the last couple of years, maybe you changed jobs several times. You're worried about how this looks on your resume. And family and friends talk about your being "unstable." After all, isn't staying in a job for a long time a sign of maturity?

Why this happens:

■ Sometimes job changes are in your best interest and sometimes they are not. If you're starting on a career track where one job leads to another and another, you may be moving each time you quickly master a step. You may find you're moving upward with increases in pay, status, and responsibility.

This will tend to happen when you're in a growing field and you have a visionary picture of where you want to go. This means, of course, that you are a big picture kind of person. You probably have a dream, one that both motivates you and urges you on toward completion.

- If you're a bright, creative person who tires quickly of any job you master, you will more than likely move on to a job from which you can learn. However, it is also possible that the pain of remaining static is so great that you quit before you have something else.

- You may get easily bored in jobs with a lot of repetition or where there's little chance for creativity or ingenuity. As a result, you feel stressed and *have* to move. This tends to happen when you have the kind of brain that likes stimulation and can process information and experiences quickly. Again, you may move responsibly or without thought, depending upon the amount of training you've had to accommodate the way in which your brain is constructed. (See Escaping Boredom, p. 239.)

- Of course, it's always possible that you have to move on because you can't get along with people, have authority issues (see Displacing Your Temper onto Others, p. 113), have an issue with addiction, or are unable to handle the job responsibly.

What not to do:

Do not automatically assume there is something wrong with you because you don't stick with a job for a long period of time.

What to do:

1. Look carefully at the reasons you change jobs. Are you moving because it is in your best interest?

2. Begin to sort through the changes you've made job-wise, by listing the jobs you've had and the reasons you've left. You can do this on paper, in your mind, or talking to someone else. You must be absolutely honest with yourself.

3. Check to see if you have a big picture in your mind, one that reflects where you're headed career-wise. Ask yourself if you have a dream or a vision you'd like to fulfill. Is that what drives you?

4. Now check to see which of your job moves has brought you closer to the completion of your goal. If each has, you can relax about the changes you've made.

5. Every single change may not have turned out to be to your benefit. That does not necessarily mean you have a problem. Ask yourself what you learned from any ill-fated change. Do you sense you made a mistake? What did you learn from that error, and how are you using that information now?

6. Note whether you've made the same mistake several times. That's a sign you need help with a pattern that's *not* in your best interest. Be brutally honest with yourself. What do you need to fix in yourself? You may need to seek consultation or counseling to get past this speed bump in your path.

7. If you get bored with jobs, you are either underemployed, doing a job with lower expectations than you are capable of meeting, need more education so you can get a more challenging job, or are in the wrong kind of job.

8. If you get easily bored, consider a job where the assignment continually changes. Some likely candidates include jobs with trouble-shooting assignments or creative design (in any field), or a job with regular new assignments such as patent law, counseling, or custom building.

9. If you are underemployed, you either need to go back to school, get additional training, or invent a new job that requires you to learn a lot

on your own. For example, if you've been a physician's assistant but keep job hopping because you get tired of the job, you may need to become a physician so you are freed of the limitations your training has placed on you. If you've been in the building trades but are tired of going from job to job where you do the same thing over and over, you may want to start your own business or design a building product for which you handle the marketing.

10. If you job hop because you can't do the job, you need to look at your initial choice of jobs and seek one that fits you better.

11. If you job hop because you lose your temper, have a chemical dependency problem, or can't get along with people, you need counseling to get your emotions and your behavior under control.

What makes this hard to do:

The hardest part of remedying job hopping is being honest with yourself about the reasons for changes. Be sure that what you're doing is truly in your best interest.

ESCAPING BOREDOM

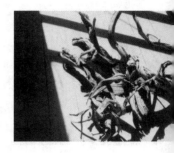

IS BOREDOM ONE OF THE GREATEST FEARS YOU FACE?

You remember how you hated school for as long as you can remember. There were so many assignments that bored you to such an extent that you refused to do them. As soon as you knew you could do the assignment, you got bored. It's the same on the job. You begin to feel so bad, you can't get yourself to continue. You *have* to quit. In school, it meant your grades weren't very good for a long time, even though you tested out pretty well. Now it means you're not making the career progress you hoped you would.

When you think about being a responsible adult, your greatest fear is that you will get stuck in a boring job. And now, here you go again. You've mastered your trade and wonder "What's next?"

Why this happens:

- When you have a quick-processing, big picture mind, you rapidly understand what's happening. You may not need to hear all the words in a sentence or see all the steps of something to know the outcome. Unlike people whose brains are constructed in a detail-oriented, step-by-step way—people who require all the details before the big picture comes together for them—you see whole patterns immediately.

- You love the feeling of newness. It makes you feel good, almost high. It brings great zest to your life. There's nothing wrong with this, though those who don't understand some-times think of newness as an addic-tion. It's only an addiction if it con-trols your life in a way that causes you trouble or is used to cover feel-ings with which you don't want to deal. A healthy love of new chal-lenges can provide you with an interesting life with quality advance-ment.

- Boredom is an indicator that you're doing something that doesn't fit you.

- It can mean you're wasting time.

That saps your life energy and shuts you off from experience, which feels bad when you're a lively, creative, curious person.

What not to do:

Do not try to force yourself to ignore your feelings of boredom.

What to do:

1. Pay attention to the messages and function of boredom and steer your life's course accordingly.

2. Review your feelings of boredom from previous years. Ask yourself, under what circumstances did they occur? What were you doing or not doing?

3. Review the times in your life, includ-ing the present time, when you felt zestful and boredom-free. What were you doing? You'll learn a lot about your needs and life path by tackling these questions.

4. Ask yourself if you have a dream. Ask if you get bored when you're not following it or some other special interest.

5. Ask whether you use activity and change to soothe feelings of boredom. When you feel good as a result, do you make constructive use of that energy, propelling yourself toward a goal of your choosing or toward your dream? Or do you use the high to escape from dealing with feelings or situations that need attention? The answer to these questions will tell you whether you have an addiction to change or can use signs of boredom creatively as a guide for constructive living.

6. When others fear you're being irresponsible because you make changes when you're bored, check within yourself and consider the work you've done. Then you'll know whether to ignore their concern or take it to heart.

If you honestly feel the accusation doesn't fit, tell the person, "Thank you for your concern. I'll take responsibility for any changes I make." Of course, you must then follow through responsibly.

7. Check to see how you handle situations in which you become bored. Ask, "Do I bolt, leaving a mess of unfinished business behind me? Do I face my commitments and responsibly take steps to extricate myself, such as giving notice on the job rather than walking out? Do I have a dream, plan, or goal in mind that I want to follow? Can I use feelings of boredom to determine whether I'm on the path to my dreams and goals or have gotten off my path?"

8. Use boredom constructively to guide you to the style of life that fits you, while acting respectful to those around you.

What makes this hard to do:

You may think you *should* remain in
certain situations even though they bore
you. But if you stay, you will struggle,
unable to live authentically in relation
to your true self.

FINDING JOBS THAT FIT

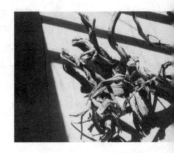

DO YOU KNOW WHAT KIND OF JOB FITS YOU?

You are a salesperson who loves to sell directly to people. You have a friend who loves computers and keeps telling you that you ought to computerize your business, selling over the Internet so you can make more money. The thought of sitting all day in front of a computer screen makes your stomach hurt. You see his enthusiasm. You know he's trying to help you, and what he says makes sense. *Everyone* says computers are the way of the future. But you keep resisting.

You wonder why he likes computers and you don't. You worry you're making a big mistake. Maybe you ought to *make* yourself be more involved with them. Selling to one person at a time is certainly slower.

Why this happens:

- You must realize that not all people, no matter what their brainstyle, have similar interests, skills, and personalities.

- As a direct salesperson, you may be in a job that makes excellent use of your brainstyle and personality.

After all, that's why you are good at what you do. You are in a right fit for someone who needs a high level of physical activity. Your ability to do more than one thing at a time and to express the naturally outgoing person you are is an asset.

- Others often inadvertently make suggestions that fit them without realizing that all people aren't made the same way. If you are not drawn to technical things, that's a sure sign that technical things aren't compatible with the way you are made. It doesn't matter how much money someone, somewhere is making or how many predictions say a particular job is the way the marketplace is going. If you don't like it, you'll feel miserable trying to do it.

What not to do:

Do not try to do what someone else does just because the person thinks his or her way is *the* way.

What to do:

1. Scrutinize your feelings and interests, noting what attracts and repels you.

2. Be sure to look at careers that not only take your style of brain construction into account, but that also support your temperament, personality, and interests.

3. Thank anyone who makes suggestions to you, and tell them you are carefully studying your options.

4. Then do not discuss your quest with anyone who isn't able to look at options through your eyes rather than their own. This is a skill that only some people have. It's precious. Only share with those who leave you feeling enthusiastic, positive, and hopeful about *yourself* and *your* future.

5. Give yourself permission to follow a career track that you love, one that excites you and allows you to be who you are.

Succeeding at Work

6. Take an inventory of times and situations in your life when you were truly happy. Ask yourself what you were doing.

7. Take a similar inventory of times and situations when you were unhappy, bored, or frustrated. Notice when your performance was lackluster and you resisted getting out of bed in the morning.

8. Get to know yourself well.

9. If you're offered a job change or promotion, look carefully at the requirements of the new setting to find out if they fit you. Often, promotions in a company can mean a change from something that fits you to something that is a complete misfit. Preferably try out the change before you commit to the job. This is like trying on a suit of clothes before buying it. If this is not possible, ask lots of questions about what you'll actually be doing, how you'll be doing it, and how you'll be evaluated.

10. Do not be blinded by offers of increased status and money. Though tempting, you must stay true to yourself and what you feel is important.

11. Think for yourself. Though the person offering you the position may have been around longer and has more status than you, you know more about yourself, your innate strengths, weaknesses, and preferences as they are dictated by your brain construction. You must take responsibility in this area.

12. If you get in a job that ends up not being a good fit for you, don't wait for things to crumble around you. Immediately go to your boss and ask for help solving the situation. Be willing to leave the job in good graces. There's no disgrace in owning up to being a poor match for a particular situation. You will be admired for your keen observation and honesty.

View from the Cliff

13. Take your values and courage in your hands and do the kind of work that fits you.

14. Find or create a personal cheering squad that knows and values you as a person the way you are.

What makes this hard to do:

You will need to remain strong within yourself. Many people will fail to understand what you're doing and why you're doing it. Surround yourself with supporters who believe in your ability to find your own answers.

IMPLEMENTING YOUR DREAM

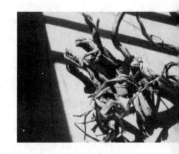

DO YOU FEAR YOU'LL NOT BE ABLE TO REACH YOUR DREAM JOB?

You've always had dreams. As long as you were in school, you figured you'd get to the place in life where you would be able to make a difference, maybe even a big difference. But now you're not sure if that was just wishful thinking. Maybe you've been overrating yourself.

"What makes you think," you wonder, "that you're someone special?" You did pretty well in school, but certainly didn't graduate at the top of your class.

You're a fairly talented speaker, good with people, and you are able to network effectively. You see things you'd like fixed in society. You know how you'd like things done, but you feel you surely are not a big enough person to be able to be effective.

You've spent time exploring so you can find your dream job. You now feel confident that you know what direction you want to go. But your next step requires you to make your dream a tangible reality.

One acquaintance suggests you start your own business. "Step one," she says.

"Create a five-year plan, including a budget." Your heart sinks. Another person stresses that you need to go back to school and get another degree. Again your body rebels as your stomach tightens and your head spins. You feel like crying. It's as if your dream is being shattered, torn away from you. You wonder if the whole dream thing was a waste of time.

Why this happens:

■ For people with a creative, kinesthenic, visionary style of brain construction, the skills required to get through school are usually quite different from those upon which success after school depends. So you may be creatively brilliant, a great leader, a superb producer/networker, inventor, or troubleshooter/fixer, but have bland grades from your formal studies. You probably also have learned a lot outside of school on your own and through experience.

■ You've not realized any of your

dreams and don't even know where to begin. But you must realize that focusing on your talents and then finding ways to implement them takes time, experience, know-how, and courage.

■ Finding and deciding which talents you want to make use of to reach your goal is a big job. Your talents can be specific, such as musical or artistic. They may be in the area of fixing or designing things or making friends. They can also be more complex, using multiple smaller skills. You may have the ability to problem-solve, be inventive, entrepreneurial, or able to network people, bringing them together for teamwork. Your talent may be in reading other people or managing details, being empathetic or psychic, leading others, or being a caregiver.

■ Talent-based skills do not necessarily show up when you are young, especially if you do okay in school. You may not find them until later in your life. The more complex the talent or set of talents you possess, the longer it may take you to find them and use them.

- If you tend to be a big picture person who likes variability and multitasking, you may become quite frustrated with traditional job roles. You may also job hop, failing to stick to one thing for very long. Even so, you could be heading to your dream even if you don't realize that's what you're doing. You must ultimately realize you can put together the experiences you absorb from each job.

- If you have a sense, however, of "specialness" but are also frustrated, you probably haven't yet synthesized the elements that must come together for you on your life pathway. Remember, though, you wouldn't feel special if you weren't.

- Finding your dream path is only step

one. There are many steps involved in implementing it. And there are many ways to take those steps. There is always a path that fits the way your brain is constructed. Living your dream is a process that can take the rest of your life. You can't know all the steps at first because many will unfold only as you move forward and increasingly see new options from which to choose.

- Anytime you get physical reactions to plans you've made so that you feel bad, know you're trying to do something in a way that isn't right for you. Similarly, if you have a negative reaction to a suggestion about how to proceed, it may be the wrong path for you to follow.

- Also, if you're trying to implement a dream—a dream that you arrived at through your feelings—you must manifest the dream by using your feelings. To switch to trying to implement it with strategic, linear thinking means you are scrambling for approval. Stay with the one that brought you to the dance. Be consistent with the process that works for you.

What not to do:

Do not discount your feeling of specialness or let anyone tell you that you ought not to try to live out your heart's feelings.

What to do:

1. Follow your interests and desires, synthesizing your talents so you become all you have ever dreamed of becoming.

2. Give yourself time to be introspective.

3. Keep a journal or somehow record your day and night dreams and your visions. Note interests to which you are drawn and those experiences that turn you off.

4. Review what you've done without judging it. For example, let's say you were involved in a venture that got you into trouble. Rather than discounting the whole experience as one big mistake to be wiped off your life experience slate, review what you liked about it. Note what you hoped for and what excited you.

   Then pay attention to what went wrong. What were you hoping for that didn't work? Did you try to go too fast or want too much too soon? Were you trying to skim corners or did you fail to be totally honest? Did you stop believing in yourself, run into obstacles you didn't know how to solve, run out of money, or trust people who turned out to be unreliable?

5. Look for patterns in what worked for and against you.

6. Search for people whose lives you admire. Ask why you admire them. What did they do that you like? Look

at the patterns in their lives as much as the specific things they did.

7. Notice what you cannot keep yourself from doing. You'll repeatedly go back to activities or interests that are right for you. Be careful not to judge yourself at this time, leaving out activities or things that you feel or have been told are "foolish," "childish," or should be relegated to the category called "hobby."

8. Now let your mind and heart soar. Just suppose that you actually can become anything you want to become.

9. Once you've arrived at a dream choice or choices, all you have to do for now is take one step. That first step may be simple or complex. If the first step is clear, then just take it. More often, though, you may need to spend time looking at a number of ways you might proceed. Many very diverse pathways will lead to your goal. Your job now is to decide which one to take next.

10. In deciding which path to use to proceed toward your goal, again listen to the feelings within yourself. Watch your reaction to suggestions from others or even to the so-called sensible voices from within. Let yourself meditate, then ask, "What's my next step?" (See Creating in Your Mind, p. 254.)

11. Ask, "How can I get these skills?" Watch and listen for an answer to all your questions. Note who calls or crosses your path. Pay attention to any interest that you start thinking about. Even notice if you are drawn to a book, including fiction, or a play or a weekend activity. Though what you're attracted to may not make sense on the surface, it'll fit perfectly into your total plan.

12. Ask, "How can I get these skills? Can I get what I need informally?" Look

around for people you know who have these skills. The people don't necessarily need to be close to you.

13. If schooling is involved, look at various ways to get that training. If credentials are needed and you feel overwhelmed about getting them or simply don't want to, do one of two things. Look for a way to practice your dream in a nontraditional way. Avoid steps that are particularly repugnant to you. Or, alternately, see if you can acquire the training and subsequent credential in a way that you can manage. (See Returning to College, p. 87.)

14. For example, if you want to help people who are elderly but the idea of getting a degree in gerontology or counseling or social work worries you, look at alternative ways to reach your goal. You might start your own business. As a businessperson, you don't need a degree. You might go into partnership with someone who has the required degree or certificates so you can do what you do well and that person meets the legal requirements.

Or, on a different track, you might host a television or radio show about and for older people. You could create plays and tour to places where older people live, putting on shows. You might include retirement home residents in the plays. You could lead elders on tours or design interiors or clothing or sports equipment for older people. How about fundraising or ministering to the elderly? Your choices of ways to work with the elderly are endless.

15. If you cringe at the thought of doing a business plan, don't do it. If the idea of a budget overwhelms you, set it aside for now. Later, when money becomes an issue for you to grow, you will notice the right person to help you learn what to do. Or you'll find a partner to take over the job.

Succeeding at Work

253

Or you'll be ready to face the budget yourself.

16. Ask yourself if you dare put your dreams out into the world to become a reality. If you can't, ask why. Whose voice do you hear in your mind, saying, "Oh, come on! Who do you think you are?" From where are the limitations coming that you are bumping into? They were learned, you know.

17. Realize that subsequent steps to making your dream a reality may take time. Make that time enjoyable. Learn a lot, try a lot, and be sure to affirm the way in which you work, honoring your styles of creation and implementation. Be flexible.

18. Don't stop unless you truly have a change of heart, but do take breaks.

19. Enjoy the journey.

What makes this hard to do:

Too often we are taught that dreams belong to childhood or there is a standard way of doing things. We give up our dreams, figuring that they are foolish. Or we forfeit our dreams because the way we were trying to achieve them didn't work. Instead, brush off a dream, go back to the drawing board, and try another pathway toward the fulfillment of it. Resist being seduced by the approval of others.

CREATING IN YOUR MIND

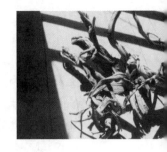

DO YOU OFTEN HAVE CREATIVE INSIGHTS, THOUGHTS, AND SOLUTIONS IN YOUR MIND WITHOUT PLANNING TO?

You are telling someone how to do something and you find yourself explaining more than you realized you knew. You have become so absorbed in your task that it actually grows before your eyes as new insights and angles appear creatively and spontaneously. You enjoy this process and the results. Even when you prepare ahead of time, you may let go of all that preparation and shift to an inner process as you begin to work.

Sometimes solutions to creative or work problems pop into your mind exactly when you need them. And often, if you ask yourself how to proceed with a project, the answer almost immediately appears. These solutions may take the form of movies or stage plays that play out before your mind's eye.

Why this happens:

- The True You is a big picture person who can draw from an infinite resource of potential bits of information within your brain. Your strength is in the relationships and processes between things. So your mind naturally tries out various details in different combinations and instantly recognizes those that please you or fit a situation. You can count on this process to fit the form or outline of an assignment even though you don't purposely *think* about it.

■ You are capable of multitasking. You can think of more than one thing at the same time, as a mental juggler. You are simultaneously able to keep a task or question in mind while working on the solution or answers. You listen to yourself as you proceed, integrating what you feel inside your mind with what you experience outside yourself, moving back and forth between the inner and outer experiences.

■ You sense rhythm well and are readily able to move from one thought to another without losing track of the various strands of the rhythm. You continuously sense them. This has a

lot to do with being an analog processor of information who has strong rhythmic intelligence.

■ You become so absorbed in what you're doing that you take on its language and follow the direction it takes you rather than superimposing your own structure on the task, thus limiting its potential growth. You *become one* with the task—a very Zen way of being.

■ Because of your style of brain construction, you can count on it to produce solutions to problems by simply introducing the problem and then letting go to allow a solution to present itself. You don't have to purposely "think it through." In fact, such purposeful thought can block successful outcomes from your style of problem-solving. You simply need to let *your way* do its job out of your conscious awareness.

What not to do:

Do not discount your inner process or judge it to have less value than more mechanistic or linear processes. Do not try to work from a tight plan that leaves no room for creative thought to emerge.

What to do:

1. Learn to use the style of working and creating that is the way of The True You.

2. Know that your way of handling information and finding answers is a tangible process with which you are blessed by virtue of solid, real brain construction. It's only a variation within the realm of human physiological potential.

3. Rejoice in your wonderful skills.

4. To learn to use your special thinking skills, practice being aware of what you're feeling as you proceed in a task. Pay attention to the situations where your creative thinking skills emerge. Compare those situations and note how and when they are strongest. Note analogies that pop into your mind. Pay attention to your prior state of mind and your level of comfort with the environment in which you find yourself. Notice your comfort with the types of people you're around when you become most creative.

5. Note what you can do to replicate or create states of mind in the future that please you. Work that is open ended and free of rigid requirements is likely to elicit your creativity. Environments that you like will more readily spawn creative achievement on your part. You are likely to find that warm, receptive, open-minded, creative people encourage your flowing productions.

6. Keep as much track of your experiences as any researcher does. This does not mean that you have to create a linear database on paper. But it

does mean that you create a mental recall system. When something you do doesn't fit into the schema that has begun to emerge in relation to your creative activity, question it. find out what is different from when something does fit. You'll figure out the differences, and they will end up making good sense to you. And you'll have learned more about yourself.

7. Give yourself permission to move in directions your senses draw you toward, rather than trying to purposely figure out what the next step *should* be.

8. Be careful of losing belief in your process. Suppose one day you aren't feeling well. Or maybe someone purposely or inadvertently pressures you into working in a more linear fashion than is right for you, and you get off track. Your creativity bites the dust and you wonder if you can count on it. That undermines your confidence in yourself and pulls your focus from your inner process to an external one.

Reassure yourself that your way does work. Get quiet. Ask your inner self to again show you the way, and you will find that your unique guidance system reasserts itself. You'll again see your mental pictures and have your spontaneous insights and solutions.

9. Be cautious about whom you talk with in relation to the way you work. Many people may not have the brain construction to work in the way that you do or even understand it. Unfortunately, they may believe that their way is the superior or the right way. Their approach can make you feel unnecessarily unsure of yourself.

10. Do not hesitate to back off from a path that is not producing or for which you have no enthusiasm.

11. Try a new direction or new angle

whenever you want, whether it makes logical sense or not. It *will* end up working for you.

12. If your creative mind works too fast for comfort, check your environment to be sure you're not feeding your mind too much stimulation. This can happen when you get talking to another creative person or are working on a team.

13. Reduce the stimulation that surrounds you. This may mean you need to go off by yourself to work for a while.

14. Consider putting yourself on a schedule and cut out extraneous activities when you are on a creative roll. This may mean letting the dishes go or the lawn grow an inch higher. It sure means to avoid problem-solving and brainstorming meetings or discussions.

15. You may also find your mind works

overtime for emotional reasons, if you have a hidden emotional agenda. Doubt about what you are doing or guilt that you're doing something wrong will cause undue stress.

16. Deal with your emotional stress before proceeding with your project agenda. If you're feeling doubt, ask where it's coming from. From whom did you learn it? Then take your courage in hand, take a stand, returning the doubt to its original source. Then follow your commitment.

    If guilt has intruded, also recall from whom you learned it. Take your power back as you revisit the value system you wish to live by at this time. (See Deciding What to Do, p. 269.)

17. If you have multiple creative, imaginative scenarios spinning in your head, make a list of the various projects and scenarios. Then make a folder for each.

18. Pick one to focus on now. It doesn't matter which one you choose. Let your heart be your guide.

19. Promise yourself you'll work with each project in turn, *one at a time.*

20. Go to work, paying attention to the project you've chosen.

21. When other ideas intrude into your thinking, write them down and put them into the folder where they belong or make a new folder for new ideas. Do not pursue the ideas further *at this time.*

22. Realize that you'll never run out of ideas. And know you'll never totally lose an idea. Even if you don't use it in its present form, it will recycle to reappear as a part of another idea. You will not suffer a loss.

23. Enjoy the wonderful mind that is a part of The True You.

What makes this hard to do:

Western culture tends to judge thinking styles, placing them into preferred categories as if there is a single way to look at things. Moving into the "flow" or process of how something works means you may have to go against the grain.

Generally, fear that you won't pick the right project also makes it hard to trust your creative thinking process. Such fear may slow you from making the choice of which project/idea/direction to pursue. In reality, it doesn't matter which one you choose. Basically you'll end up being you, expressing your creative self, and creating something that will be wonderful and will please you.

You will have to learn to believe in yourself and surround yourself with supportive people.

View from the Cliff

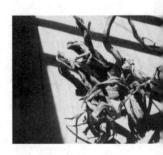

SUCCEEDING AS A CREATIVE EMPLOYEE

DO YOU HAVE TROUBLE WORKING FOR PEOPLE WHO REQUIRE YOU TO DO THINGS THEIR WAY?

You have always been a creative person. Your last boss gave you a lot of freedom to choose projects to your liking. You had creative freedom to follow your interests. Sometimes you worked non-stop when you were feeling especially productive, and other times you kicked back when you didn't feel like working. You've always worked hard, been highly productive, and made a lot of money for the company. You've never missed a deadline.

Now you have a new boss who has his own ideas about how things ought to be done. He's begun to assign specific projects to employees along with time-lines to follow. He wants you there *on time* and requires you to stay even if you are not having a productive day. He actually wants employees to leave when he leaves. Though you have less work to do, you have begun to hate your job. You've started to avoid work, take long lunches, and use your sick leave and vacation time. You daydream and can hardly get yourself to be civil to cowork-ers, much less your boss. You've tried talking to him, to no avail. You're seriously considering quitting.

Why this happens:

- Your mental style fit your previous supervisor's management style. As a creative person, you are guided from within, marching, as they say, to your own drum. You are a responsible person who is more than willing to take control of any work project in which you believe.

- Because you have an inner guiding light that is sensitively attuned to your creative mood, one that is intricately interwoven to your heart's desires, you always know what fits you. And that makes you feel good. You also know what is not part of your innate life's agenda. Trying to work on something that doesn't fit you makes you feel awful, enough so that you may feel you can't stand it another minute.

- You have a wonderful sense of natural timing that works for you. It is uneven, causing you to work a lot one day and not much another, but you have a clear sense of project timelines. You simply don't break time up in a systematic way. That's not the way your analog-processing mind orders time. You order time by the content of what you're doing and the feelings within yourself.

- Given a problem to solve, your creative mind will immediately go to work finding a solution. You will move to your own rhythm. Probably you'll be keeping the end goal in sight throughout.

  But when someone requires you to use their steps, their rhythm, and their timing, you are likely to not only dislike the task, but fail to do the task well. As a responsible person, you will sense the lack of fit and probably become angry and experience a high level of stress. As a result, you may begin to lose your commitment to your job. In turn, you will no longer be able to act responsibly, which in and of itself will cause you more stress. A vicious cycle will have been set in motion. Depression is not unlikely, and your self-esteem will suffer.

What not to do:

Neither compromise your mental health nor allow yourself to act in a way that makes you less than proud and happy with yourself.

What to do:

1. Put yourself in a work situation that fits you and allows you to use your creativity.

2. Assess your situation. Think about the last time you were happy on the job. Check the fit of your brain construction and your personality with the duties, pacing, and creative freedom attached to the job at that time.

3. Note what's changed. Be as specific and detailed as you can. You may find that telling someone the details that surrounded any change will help you recall small bits of information that will hold the key to your understanding your situation. Ask the person listening to be on the lookout for shifts in your expression. Your feelings will reflect what started going wrong and be expressed on your face and through your body language.

4. Spend some time alone reviewing your values. Ask yourself what's important to you at this time. How do you want to lead your life? Consider whether a job is a job to supply living expenses, which is okay, or something that makes a statement about who you are. Does it reflect your talents and desires? Is it heartfelt?

5. Look practically at the commitments and obligations you have at this time. This will include family, debt, and

other involvements. Check to see the length of time you can anticipate the obligations to last. Be cautious that you don't automatically accept past decisions and current involvements as obligations that are unchangeable.

For example, suppose you have lived in the same neighborhood for many years and assumed that your kids would graduate from high school there. But now that you're miserable on your job, you need to be sure that you still feel the same way about where you live, because you might need to move.

If you have a child who is a high school senior, you may decide this is definitely not a time to move. But if your kids are younger or older and perhaps are at transition times, you and your family may realize you can make a change that will be a whole lot better for you and one that will not hurt them.

6. Hold a family meeting and share what is happening to you at work. Share your feelings. Ask for observations and input from everyone, your spouse and kids alike.

7. Then decide with your spouse whether a change to something that fits you better is in order as soon as possible or whether you will make the best of the situation for the time being, promising yourself a change later. If you choose the latter, find ways to use your creativity on the job or outside of work—ways that bring you in touch with your heart and bring hope into your life.

8. If you stay with the job, look for opportunities to transfer to a different boss or ask for autonomy with regard to parts of your work.

9. Keep reminding yourself that your situation is temporary and that you will stand by your creative nature. Stay alert to opportunities that will bring you a better fit.

What makes this hard to do:

The hardest part of succeeding as a creative employee is failing to believe in yourself and losing hope that you'll ever feel happy and genuinely productive again. That's your battle. Rise to the occasion, and you will be happy and productive once more.

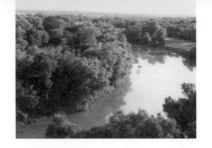

PART SIX

Epilogue

*A journey of a thousand miles must
begin with a single step.*

LAO-TZU

C. 604–C. 531 B.C.

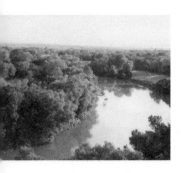

Throughout View from the Cliff, *I've shared much of what I've personally learned and professionally observed over many years.* The more I've learned, the more I've come to realize the importance of honoring human diversity, for that builds the broadest foundation for healthy living in a wholesome society. As each of us plays the role we are best suited to play, we add a unique ingredient to the mix of any achievement, dream, or goal we value.

The wiser I've become, the more I have come to value the intrinsic potential each of us has within ourselves to know what is right for us. Truly, no one else knows as well what fits us as we do, so we can use our natural talents and skills to their maximum. Yet I've repeatedly seen disconnection from that inner knowing as we are taught what we need *to do, how we* should *be, or what we* ought *to want.*

Often shared in well-meaning ways, these *shoulds* and oughts *break the connection we have with our true selves. The True You is the vehicle that knows how to bring your potential to its peak level of performance.*

Finally, the more self-aware I've become and the stronger I've grown emotionally, the more I realize the effect each of us can have on the direction our lives take. As we believe, so we create. These are not empty words. The power of belief to affect outcomes is only beginning to be understood and acknowledged. We are a long way from harnessing that power. And we each have much emotional work to do to get beyond the self-imposed limitations created by our fears, doubts, and disbelief in this power that is available to each of us. But we are learning to use the power of belief for the valuable expression of our true selves.

To achieve the success that benefits both ourselves and the society in which we live, we must fully honor our true selves, scrupulously engaging, whenever possible, in what fits our makeup: our style of brain construction, our personalities, and our interests and heartfelt desires.

We must gently and knowingly encourage the parts of our behavior and emotions that have been hurt, healing our wounded selves.

And, when necessary, we must make sure we do not further wound ourselves as our accommodating selves strive to live and learn in today's world.

I'd like to end this book with two additional exercises. One is entitled "Deciding What to Do." It highlights the reasons it's hard to honor what we want, caught instead in the trap of trying to do what we think we should do. And it gives

you steps to consider that will allow you to marry your thinking with your desire, to respect and express The True You by doing what you want to do, not what you should do.

The second and final exercise, "Building a Life According to What You Believe," will guide you in relation to enhancing your ability to use the power inherent in what you believe. Then, as you choose, you can purposely create a life of your own making by becoming aware of what you believe and using that belief to create the outcomes you desire.

In View from the Cliff, *I leave you with that which I've garnered from my journey. I intend for it to be helpful and empowering to you. I also encourage you to take only what fits you. Honor your own timing and only select the parts to which you are drawn. Above all, know that I respect and value The True You. With confidence, I release my words into your care.*

Epilogue

DECIDING WHAT TO DO

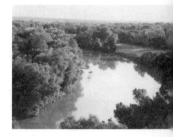

DO YOU HAVE TROUBLE DECIDING TO LET YOURSELF DO WHAT YOU'D *REALLY* LIKE TO DO?

Maybe you are trying to decide whether to go back to work or continue to stay home full-time with your child. Or maybe you're wondering whether to become an artist, but reason tells you to become a teacher. Perhaps your heart desires to fly airplanes, but your partner wants you to stay safely on the ground.

Every time you think about your dreams and desires, you start out feeling wonderful, hopeful, and enthusiastic about your life. You feel willing to work hard and are motivated to do whatever is necessary to reach your goal. But then *reality* sets in. Either someone with whom you share your dreams says something to the effect of "Come on now. Get a grip! You know you should be responsible. You can't make a living *that* way." Or you might hear, "Don't be so selfish. Your child needs you." Or you hear your partner saying, "You have a family now. You should grow up and quit playing with toys."

Guilt and fear paralyze you. Though you may feel trapped, depressed, and generally miserable, it will take a lot of personal power to stand up against what you think you should do.

Why this happens:

- You are being swayed by what you think you *should* do rather than following the lead of what you *want* to do. This means your behavior is driven by "shoulds." A "should" is a belief, that is, something you were *taught* at an earlier time by someone else. A belief's power lies in the fact that you learned it when you were very young and dependent on those around you who were guiding your behavior. Because of this powerful, early learning—learning that is often forgotten by all of us when we grow older—we tend to think what we believe is *the only way* to think. That is why beliefs are hard to change.

- The words *should* and *ought* continue to carry a strong legacy from early years, so much so that you tend to revert to feeling dependent when they are used.

- When you do something you don't think you *should* do, you will tend to feel *guilty*. When you do something you don't *want* to do, you'll feel *resentful*. Either way, you feel bad.

- As a result, the *shoulds* control your life. But they also cheat you of your life. They may pull you away from acting in behalf of The True You. They may separate you from what you love. They control your actions, driving you to act in ways that may not be good for The True You.

- When what you have been taught doesn't fit you naturally, you will become conflicted and unable to know what to do. You will have a hard time making decisions. This is because there is a strong drive within all of us to live in alignment with our true selves. This feels like *desire* and *wanting,* while a belief to the contrary contradicts that tendency.

What not to do:

Do not fail to align your belief systems with The True You.

What to do:

1. Rethink the beliefs you were taught at an earlier time so you can decide if you want to keep them or not.

2. Ask yourself what the belief is that is causing you conflict, i.e., "What do I think I *should* do?" For example, consider the belief "I *should* stay home with my child and do my housework."

3. Ask yourself, "From whom did I learn this belief?" Watch for snippets of thoughts, memories, mental pictures, and conversations in your mind. They are likely to reflect the settings in which you learned the belief. You may instantly recall the exact person from whom you learned it. Or your learning may have occurred in a more subtle way as you sensed what many people around you believed, even if they never said anything directly to you.

4. Next ask yourself if you practiced the belief so you would be praised and feel accepted. Or did you adhere to the guidelines of the belief because you were afraid not to do so? Disapproval may have created feelings of fear if you are a sensitive person. Of course, you might also have been afraid of being punished if you didn't follow the dictates of the belief.

5. If you suffer from the fear of repercussions when you don't do what someone else wants, begin to build your independence and courage to stand up for what *you* think is right. Use the pronoun "I" liberally. You

might say, "*I* make decisions based on what I know about myself. *I* am in charge of myself."

6. Next check to see what new information you have obtained that you didn't have previously. For example, you now know that brain diversity affects what each individual does. You may realize that there is no *one right way* for everyone.

7. Notice the effects of trying to do something that doesn't fit you but that you feel you *should* do. Perhaps feelings of resentment come to mind. Or guilty feelings or depression or anger. Simply note them. You will come to realize that you don't have to continue to feel any of these when you rework your belief system to fit The True You *while* you continue to live a caring, responsible life.

8. Now decide what you want to believe. You may either adopt a new belief or continue the previous one. If you continue the previous one, it now is one that belongs to you because you've thought through it. It's no longer a *should.* You've made it your own by choosing it with your adult mind and heart working in unison.

Or you may decide you want to modify your previous belief based on the new information you've obtained. For example, using the example of the young mother, you might decide you are going to give yourself permission to get a job doing what you love because the other course simply doesn't work for you. You become creative about how to use your time with your child. You make sure you have a job with flexibility so you can be available to your child at special times.

And you decide to spend some of your wages on housecleaning services. You might even decide to take on a few extra hours so you can pay for yard work, too.

Again referring to the young mother, the nice part about her work with her values is that she gets what fits her while still being a responsible person. And her child gets a fulfilled parent who can teach her child how to also live up to his or her natural self.

What makes this hard to do:

Because beliefs are initially learned when we are very young and dependent and have black and white thinking, we tend to feel they are cast in concrete. We may not question them, much less think to change them, even though our thinking has matured to take on the gray cast of adult life.

BUILDING A LIFE ACCORDING TO WHAT YOU BELIEVE

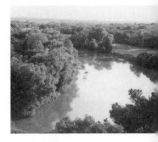

DO YOU STRUGGLE TO BELIEVE POSITIVELY ABOUT YOUR TRUE SELF?

All your life you've felt different, not performing as well as other people in certain areas. You've tried to be well rounded, but no matter how hard you try, you fail in some things while succeeding in others. You wonder if there is something wrong with you because of your failures.

You almost wish there was because then you would have an excuse for why you can't do some things better. Maybe then you could *be fixed*. But you also feel sad thinking you might have something *wrong* with you because thinking about it takes your time and attention away from enjoying the things you love about yourself. You feel confused.

Why this happens:

■ You may have learned you're okay no matter what your race, religion, sex, sexual preference, age, or interests. These all fall under the rubric of diversity. But diversity in brainstyles has not yet achieved equivalent status.

■ In a society that has historically struggled with diversity, any group of people that is not like the model held up as the preferred way to be is considered inadequate until that group of people refuses to be seen as lesser any longer.

■ Any preferred model is a mental construct, an illusion that one kind of person is perfect.

■ But every attribute of brainstyle has strengths and weaknesses. Every strength has a down side and every weakness has an up side.

■ Some of your characteristics that have been shaped by your style of brain construction will be favored by the cultural model under which you live. Others won't, no matter what your unique style.

■ In reality, there is absolutely nothing *wrong* with you, no matter what your style of brain construction. To the degree to which you have been constantly placed in environments that don't fit you, taught in ways that don't fit your brainstyle, and had expectations made of you that fail to take brainstyle diversity into account, you will have been wounded. You may *feel* there is something wrong with you when, in reality, you've simply been hurt by living in a misfitting environment. The True You is just fine.

■ The myth that there is something wrong with people who have different styles of brain construction was passed on to our generation and is being passed to future generations. However, what we believe, we create. We now have a chance to stop wasting human potential for ourselves and for our children and our children's children as diversity of brainstyle is recognized for what it is.

What not to do:

Do not believe you are anything less than wonderful *as you are.*

What to do:

1. Accept the power you have to create

a self-image that is positive and yields constructive results for you and the world around you. Honor the unique attributes that make you up.

2. Remember, the way in which you view yourself affects not only how you feel about yourself, but how and what you are able to do in your life. It affects your behavior.

3. Remember, you have the power to create a positive self-image by accepting the unique combination of brainstyle attributes you possess. You can affirm this by saying, "I create a positive self-image of myself. I see myself as fine, just the way I am made."

4. Become self-aware of your brainstyle without judging it.

5. Become aware of the learning and working and living environments that suit the way in which your brain is constructed.

6. Affirm your desire to fit into those environments. You can say, "I find the environments in which to learn, work, and live—environments that naturally fit me."

7. Support and nurture parts of yourself that have been hurt because of a lack of understanding of brain diversity. Identify behavior that is the result of a poor self-belief and target it for change. Counseling, hypnotherapy, and/or prayer may be useful in doing this.

8. When you are ready, forgive those who judged and hurt you because of the way your brain is constructed, for they knew and know not what they do.

    You do not need to rush this step. Take your time.

9. Build bridges to environments that don't fit you without judging yourself or the environments. Say, "I build a bridge to any environment in which I find myself, even though I

and my environment utilize different brainstyles."

10. Consider mentoring others so they can see themselves as valuable while teaching them to effectively use the skills their brainstyles provide them.

11. Refuse to accept current terms that *pathologize* your *condition.*

12. Consider becoming active in changing the perception of people who have brainstyle attributes that do not fit the standardized social model. This means working to see that every child receives an education that fits him or her. Equal educational opportunity for all people regardless of brain diversity is critical. Equal opportunity means that a person's ability to do a job or show what he or she knows is assessed in ways that reflect his or her style of brain con-struction. It means standing up against professionals who say differently.

As the perception of the public is heightened, the major diversity issue of the twenty-first century will be successfully put to rest as all styles of brain construction are equally honored and allowed to function.

13. Learn the language of those with a different style of brain construction from yours.

14. Learn how to team up with those who are different so that goals can be reached and growth achieved in balanced ways.

What makes this hard to do:

Changing beliefs is one of the hardest jobs anyone can tackle.